Violence and the Brain

This being of mine, whatever it really is, consists of a little flesh, a little breath, and the part which governs.

Marcus Aurelius Antonius
Meditations

VIOLENCE *and the* BRAIN

Vernon H. Mark, M.D.

DIRECTOR, NEUROSURGICAL SERVICE, BOSTON CITY HOSPITAL; CLINICAL ASSOCIATE IN NEUROSURGERY, MASSACHUSETTS GENERAL HOSPITAL; AND ASSOCIATE PROFESSOR OF SURGERY, HARVARD MEDICAL SCHOOL, BOSTON

Frank R. Ervin, M.D.

DIRECTOR, STANLEY COBB LABORATORIES FOR PSYCHIATRIC RESEARCH, MASSACHUSETTS GENERAL HOSPITAL; PSYCHIATRIST, MASSACHUSETTS GENERAL HOSPITAL; AND ASSOCIATE PROFESSOR OF PSYCHIATRY, HARVARD MEDICAL SCHOOL, BOSTON

Medical Department

HARPER & ROW, PUBLISHERS

New York, Evanston, and London

This book is dedicated to the Neuro-Research Foundation of Boston, *whose goals for the early diagnosis and proper treatment of the violent patient parallel our own.*

 Printed in the United States of America. For information address Medical Department, Harper & Row, Publishers, Inc., 2350 Virginia Avenue, Hagerstown, Maryland 21740

First Edition

STANDARD BOOK NUMBER: 06-141698-3

LIBRARY OF CONGRESS CATALOG CARD NUMBER: 72-83610

Contents

Foreword by William H. Sweet, M.D. vii
Preface to the Third Printing xi
Preface xiii
Acknowledgments xv
Introduction 1
1 The Problem of Violence 3
2 Our Emotional Brain 13
3 Rage, Anger, and Fear 26
4 Genetic Brain Disease 47
5 Acquired Brain Disease and Violence 55
6 The Surgery of Violence 69
7 Brain Triggers for Violence 92
8 Hidden Brain Disease 112
9 The Dyscontrol Syndrome 125
10 The Either/Or Philosophy 138
11 The Relation of the Dyscontrol Syndrome to Violence in Our Society 146
12 Violence Prevention 155
Appendix I Social and Ethical Issues: Brain Surgery in Aggressive Epileptics 163
Appendix II Recent Data on Case Histories 172
Index 177

Foreword

The principal thesis of this book evolves from the concept that human behavior, including violent assaultive action, is an expression of the functioning brain. It follows that one of the keys to understanding and controlling the current colossal problem of violence is to increase our knowledge of those brain mechanisms relating to emotion in general and dangerous aggression in particular. Although this seems so unassailably logical that it is not worth mentioning, it is only within the last three to four decades that we have been able to sketch the main outlines of the areas of the brain concerned with feeding, fleeing, fighting, and sexual activity—the principal types of activity having an emotional component. Along with awareness of the importance of studies of freely moving animals under controlled conditions, the essential experimental techniques have gradually emerged that have enabled us to learn the precise and often tiny areas of the brain concerned with these four types of behavior. It has been especially informative to stimulate electrically or to destroy small brain regions to delineate the zones and conditions connected with initiation or potentiation, and those for suppression, of emotional responses.

The authors of this book and I, one of their collaborators, are among the physicians who only recently have sought to apply the massive body of knowledge gleaned from experiments in animals to the problem of assaultiveness in man. Incidental observations of the site of the brain disorder in those human diseases associated with senseless violence have also proved relevant. Two major factors have deterred the medical profession from mounting sooner a full-scale effort to understand the details of the brain mechanisms related to violence of man: (1) we have assumed that the causes lie largely in the social environment, and (2) we have preferred to have nothing to do with these ill-tempered, dangerous people.

On the first score, we physicians have been content to accept the theories of those sociologists, anthropologists, economists, and psychologists who have proposed that man is an innately fighting, murderous species incessantly warring over territorial boundaries, women, and food (and drink). According to this viewpoint, the killer tendency is enhanced by broad cultural or narrow individual learning and is especially aggravated by such factors as crowding, deprivation of food and shelter, and by more complex social and economic inequalities. As we turn our gaze in the search for truth toward the facts of history, the current headlines, and finally onto the mirror of ourselves, most of us cheerlessly conclude that these hypotheses are indeed disturbingly probable. We physicians had seen little likelihood of our making a special contribution to the violence problem. Drs. Mark and Ervin, however, present a convincing case that there is a role for physicians to play in the violence problem in terms of diagnosing and treating those individuals who have focal brain disease as at least part of the cause of their unacceptable actions. Acknowledging that such people exist and treating them in no way controverts the evidence that environmental factors also play a huge role in the whole dismal picture. Indeed, the lessons learned about the way the emotional brain functions in violent individuals *with* localized brain disease may help us understand better how to teach mastery of these brain functions in violent, but nondiseased people.

On the second score, we physicians have almost all encountered, as obvious symptoms of disease, violent behavior in our patients. We have found the whole experience so disagreeable or personally threatening that virtually no physician, even in this age of intense specialization, has decided to specialize in treating violent patients. The authors of this book are among the very few exceptions to the foregoing statement in the entire world medical profession.

They have not found the going easy. The best equipped and

most distinguished hospitals do not like to admit as in-patients persons who have a known problem of violence, regardless of the cause. This is especially tragic in certain types of epilepsy, for example, in which there also is uncontrolled dangerous behavior which may occur with the same abruptness and unpredictability as the convulsive seizure. Moreover, potentially useful treatment exists both for seizures and assaultiveness, which requires hospitalization of such patients. Yet a hospital's reluctance to admit such patients is not as illogical or cruel as it might seem. Individuals with poor control of dangerous impulses are so disruptive of well-regulated hospital routines that their presence poses a threat to other patients and their attendants unless extraordinary precautions are taken.

Members of an overburdened nursing and ancillary staff may threaten resignation if their efficiency is impaired and their health or lives threatened by patients known to have injured others. This often proves to be true even in purely psychiatric hospitals. The medical director of the mental hospitals in one state has said that these violent patients frighten the other patients, that they frighten the nurses and orderlies, and that they frighten him. In most jurisdictions, the only available option is to allow these violent persons periods of freedom in society punctuated by loss of employment, automobile and other accidents, family upheaval and divorce, fines and prison sentences until such time as they commit a really heinous attack on one or more persons. More permanent incarceration in a jail or institution for the criminally insane follows, and the individual becomes a permanent drain on the public purse and a total loss to the culture.

Drs. Mark and Ervin present the evidence that there is now another option, that of providing a special institute or unit staffed not only by competent physicians but also by attendants specially trained to subdue a patient in his violent phases without significant injury to anyone involved. That tests may be developed to spot at an early stage the person with poor control of dangerous impulses is an especially appealing likelihood.

The Neuro-Research Foundation, on the basis of the work described in this book, is planning to operate such an institute devoted in substantial part to the now feasible diagnosis and treatment of persons with poor control of dangerous impulses. Its Board of Trustees, which includes Drs. Mark and Ervin, thinks that this volume has been written in a style comprehensible to any intelligent person and hopes that it will evoke helpful criticisms and significant financial and intellectual support for such a program.

WILLIAM H. SWEET, M.D., D.Sc.
Chief, Neurosurgical Service
Massachusetts General Hospital
Professor of Surgery
Harvard Medical School
Boston, Massachusetts

Preface to the Third Printing

This monograph has evoked from numerous members of the psychiatric community the criticism that it advocates indiscriminate use of psychosurgical management as a therapeutic modality in preventing violent behavior. We feel that this judgment is invidious. Our concept, set within a framework of the sociobiological theory of behavior, runs diametrically counter to the theoretical basis of political psychiatry, which has as one of its keystones that the human brain is a "tabula rasa", responding in a completely passive manner to the sociopolitical environment. This approach—a variation of the theme propounded by John Locke, eminent English political philosopher of the late 17th century—has enjoyed a recent revival in the sphere of social science. Locke's philosophy of environment-brain dualism is related to the Aristotelian concept of separation of body and psyche, a more complete discussion of which is found in Chapter 10.

The physiological observations made on Thomas's and Julia's studies (Ch. 7), together with other substantial evidence, render improbable the "tabula rasa" theory of violent behavior. Because our data contradict some of the basic doctrines of political psychiatry, our investigative group has been subjected to criticism that is ostensibly aimed at the discipline of psychosurgery. Having carried out no surgical intervention on patients with primary psychiatric disease since 1963 (see Appendix II, Mark *et al.*, Ref. 13—Operation, 1963; published 1970) and advocating rigorous control of all psychosurgical treatment, we regard this criticism both as unjustified and as a tactic designed to deflect the focus of scientific investigation from the anachronistic theories that form the basis of political psychiatry and the exclusive social causation of abnormal behavior.

Recent information supporting the stands taken in this monograph are included as addenda for the third reprinting. Appendix I is a reprint of an article which I authored for *The Hastings Center Report:* Appendix II updates several of the case histories, supplying clinical support for our sociobiologically oriented approach to the problems of violent behavior.

Vernon H. Mark, M.D.

Preface

We have written this book to stimulate a new and biologically oriented approach to the problem of human violence. The prevailing attitude of those who share the responsibility for dealing with violent individuals seems to follow two divergent pathways—pathways often closely linked with a particular philosophy. The first claims that violence is caused by a lack of effective law enforcement. The second blames social disorganization, poverty, discrimination, and the abuses of public news media—such as radio, television, newspapers and magazines—for violence. Both of these seemingly divergent views have two things in common: They advocate purely social remedies for the control of violence; and they concentrate on the perpetrators of violence as a group, making no serious effort to understand or treat the violence-prone individual.

We do not discount the importance of either of these views. But the remedies they suggest have not reduced the level of violence in our country or in the world. Even those social scientists who disdain a biological approach to what they consider an exclusively social problem will have to agree that a new point of view might be helpful. We hope that they will examine this volume without prejudice.

The material in this book is presented along traditional lines: a statement of the problem; a brief review of the structure and function of the emotional or limbic brain; a survey of the diseased states—both inherited and acquired—that can disturb limbic brain function and predispose toward violent behavior; a description of treatment—especially surgical therapy—and new findings about brain triggers and brakes that have been uncovered in the course of this therapy; a discussion of the philosophical and social responses to the challenge of violence; and a plan for a more rational approach to the violence problem—a plan that utilizes the skills of the brain scientists and clinicians. This book is not meant to supply instant answers or complete solutions to the complex problem of violence. It is meant, however, to initiate a more effective search for these answers than has been possible when the brain is ignored as the key to human behavior.

At first our intent was to write a monograph for physicians who specialize in the nervous system. But we believed the mass of clinical detail (now reflected only in the bibliography) would discourage many potential readers for whom the social implications of the book might be of value. Thus we shortened and summarized our material so that this monograph also might be read with profit by the intelligent lay reader. We hope that we have succeeded in this task, for we feel that the social-medical challenge of violence is unmistakable and the goal of a multidisciplinary approach to violence prevention is eminently worthwhile.

Boston, Massachusetts

VERNON H. MARK, M.D.
FRANK R. ERVIN, M.D.

Acknowledgments

We should like to acknowledge the support given to the research which underlies the clinical work reported in this book. We are grateful to the Department of Health, Education and Welfare—more specifically, to the National Cancer Institute, the Social and Rehabilitation Service, the National Institute of Mental Health, and the U.S. Public Health Service for the grant entitled "Injury Prevention—The Dangerous Driver" and for a career development award from the National Institute of Mental Health held by one of us (Frank R. Ervin). In addition, the Dreyfus Foundation has supported work concerning the focal application of Dilantin to the brain.

Dr. William Sweet has been both a leader and a collaborator in the various studies described in Chapters 6 through 9. It is only fair to state that without his guidance this book could never have been written. We owe a special debt to our neurological colleagues, Dr. Norman Geschwind, Dr. Robert Young, and Dr. Janice Stevens. Their collaboration and thoughtful criticism have been of inestimable value. Our psychiatric colleagues, Dr. John Lion, Dr. George Bach-Y-Rita, Dr. Carlos Climent, Dr. Mike Nelson, and Dr. Lawrence Roth greatly assisted us in working up the groups of patients described in Chapter 9. Dr. Lawrence Razavi, the cytogeneticist, gave significant help in preparing the text and bibliography for Chapter 4.

Our special thanks go to Forest Eastman, for painstakingly going over the bibliography, and to Mrs. Edith Tagrin of the Medical Art Department of the Massachusetts General Hospital for her excellent art demonstrations. Mrs. Barbara Fried labored long and hard to help us transform our usual medical jargon into language that could also be understood by the nonmedical reader. The Medical Book Department at Harper & Row, Publishers, have been particularly helpful in preparing this book for publication. Susan Shields has diligently typed draft after draft of the manuscript, aided by Cynthia Hall, Ida Stone, and Fay Burns. Elek Toth, Jim Reynolds, and Mildred Riley have given us able technical assistance in the laboratory and operating room. Any inaccuracies and inadequacies in the text, of course, remain the sole responsibility of the authors.

Finally, we are grateful to our wives, Alexandra and Pat. Bringing a book to fruition, even a small one such as this, is much easier when there is an atmosphere of congeniality and encouragement, and this was supplied in liberal portions by our wives and families.

Boston, Massachusetts

VERNON H. MARK, M.D.
FRANK R. ERVIN, M.D.

Violence and the Brain

Introduction

Human violence is the most threatening problem in our world today. And although it is a problem that is both formidable and complex, we believe that it is potentially solvable. This cautiously optimistic point of view contrasts markedly with recent public statements and articles which contain an aura of hopelessness and a feeling of despair. The proponents of these arguments state that human beings have always been violent, and that in fact, unprovoked violence is part of human nature. Or to put it more explicitly, the tendency to indulge in unprovoked violence is an instinct which every human being is born with. Further they state that the control of violence is maintained by "weak" learned behavior.

We most heartily disagree with such statements. Human beings do have instincts, but unprovoked violence is not among them. Instead, the instinct possessed by humans and represented by basic mechanisms in the central part of their brain is the instinct for *self-preservation*. And in threatening situations, this is translated by a given individual into either flight or fight—more often the former than the latter. This basic mechanism, however, can be powerfully modified by learning or environmental experience into a reaction that we would define as unprovoked violence. We believe that this translation occurs more readily in individuals with damaged or malfunctioning brains. Our evidence for this view will be presented in the subsequent chapters.

Even though violence is a widely popularized phenomenon, it is, in fact, poorly understood. For many years, it was ascribed to a faulty genetic inheritance or an evil nature. More recently environmental scientists have captured the popular imagination and public funds by ascribing violence to poverty, discrimination, to personal isolation in an increasingly fragmented society, or to a combination of these factors that produces an overwhelming sense of frustration in members of the deprived groups.

In this volume we are not going into a detailed discussion of these social causes of violence. Instead we shall focus on the relation of violence to the brain, since the brain is the storehouse of all human experience—social, cultural, and educational—and the generator of all human behavior, both peaceful and violent. We do not say that all violence is caused by people with damaged brains. We do know, however, that all behavior filters through the central nervous system, and we believe therefore that studying the relationship between the brain and violence is the best way to get to understand the mechanisms of violent behavior. We assume that these mechanisms can be identified and described, and furthermore, that some of them are related to a malfunction of the brain—a malfunction that can be tested for objectively. If we can only learn to identify those people within our society who have a low threshold for impulsive violence because they suffer from brain malfunction, we will have taken the first step toward treating these individuals; and what is more important from the public point of view, toward preventing their violent behavior.

Chapter 1

The Problem of Violence

Beware lest you lose the substance
by grasping at the shadow.

Aesop

The Dog and the Shadow

Violence is, without question, both prominent and prevalent in American life. In 1968 more Americans were the victims of murder and aggravated assault in the United States than were killed and wounded in seven-and-one-half years of the Vietnam war; and altogether almost half a million of us were the victims of homicide, rape, and assault. During the same year, an additional 60,000 Americans died and three million more were injured by automobile violence. We do not mean to indicate that the chance of death from violent causes among 200 million mainland Americans is the same as the incidence among our troops in war-torn Vietnam. But these statistics (inadequate and on the low side) do reflect a domestic scene which is far from tranquil. Many people are afraid to venture out on the city streets at night, and with good reason. Major emergency or receiving hospitals in every city of the United States have a predictable number of "Violence Victims"—people admitted daily for major surgical treatment. While it is true that we are not "at war" in Boston or Chicago, we certainly could not be described as being "at peace."

In fact, violence is one of our major public health problems. As such it has many different aspects. The aspect we are concerned with in this book is *personal* violent behavior—unwarranted and usually unprovoked acts that directly attempt to or actually do injure or destroy another person or thing. We are all too familiar with this sort of violence. In the last decade it has been highlighted by political assassinations, Whitman's multiple killings from the Texas tower, and Speck's murders. It also underlies the wanton slayings and senselessly enraged reactions of bad drivers, muggers, barroom brawlers, child beaters, and rapists who supply our newspapers with sensational copy and help make our streets, homes, cars, and airplanes unsafe. And although other animals also indulge in violent behavior, the repertoire of individual violence and the social environment within which it occurs are uniquely characteristic of the human species.

The organ of behavior is the brain, which means that in discussing violence we are actually talking about one of the ways brain function is expressed in behavior. In stressing the role of the brain, we are not denying the importance of social influences on behavior. We are well aware of the economic and social injustices that drive groups of people to riot and rebellion; the increasing sense of alienation and frustration that pervades our technological society; and the provocative accounts and depictions of violence to which we are daily exposed in papers and magazines, or on movie and television screens. Nor are we discounting the effects of education, personal history, evolutionary heritage, genetic endowment, and individual biological and psychological makeup. The fact is, however, that all these influences and events impinge on, are stored in, and are translated into behavior patterns solely by the brain—so that no matter from what point we start, we always come back to that organ's primary importance.

It is our belief that until we understand more about how brain activity is reflected in behavior, we will not fully understand what causes individual violence. However, we contend that it is possible to make a beginning, even at our present state of knowledge, in predicting and recognizing the potentially violent individual; and we intend to establish, even at our present level of technology, that it is also possible to control violent behavior in some destructive individuals. Our aim is to convince those who read this book that preventing individual violence depends on establishing cooperation and communication between brain scientists, physicians, public officials, social scientists, and geneticists. And—last but not least—it also depends on receiving the money to continue the research already begun, as well as to initiate new research programs.

As doctors, we view individual violence as a medical as well as a social problem; we have already mentioned its implications for public health and safety, but there are also two other reasons why we think it is a medical matter. First, because many of the individuals who act violently have brain diseases that can be described, diagnosed, treated, and controlled—which is to say that we believe that more often than not the kind of individual violence we are discussing is related to brain malfunction. Secondly, individuals who lose control of their anger and repeatedly attack or injure others and themselves want and need medical help, but they are not getting it. Of 150 such people we have recently seen for treatment, nearly half had been driven to attempted suicide by their despair at what they had done. All of them were aware of a sense of alienation during their periods of lost control, and felt anguished at the social and personal consequences of their acts. And all of them had gone to doctors many times before for advice and aid. Unfortunately, most physicians are not aware how often a brain abnormality may underlie violent behavior, and they are not accustomed to consider violence a medical problem. Consequently, they reject violent people as patients, dismissing them as incurable socio- or psychopaths when they should instead be looking for evidence of brain dysfuntion.

The theories about violence which focus on human nature and its interactions with environment, and our social attitudes toward criminals, law, and personal responsibility always take for granted that every individual has a normally functioning, entirely healthy brain. Most people consider brain disease to be a rare phenomenon. It is likely, however, that more than ten million Americans suffer from an obvious brain disease, and the brains of perhaps another five million have been subtly damaged (see *Appendix*). We do not mean to say that all of these brain-diseased people are violent. What we are saying is that an appreciable percentage of the relatively few individuals guilty of repeated personal violence are to be found in this 5 to 10 per cent of the population whose brains do not function in a perfectly normal way.

As we said above, the brain is the organ of behavior. Any act or state of being (i.e., behavior or thought) is a reflection of some particular mode of organization of the complex circuits of the brain. This mode of organization is determined by four things:

1. The physical structure of the brain and its chemical environment.
2. The moment-to-moment information being received by the brain from the outside world and the rest of the body.
3. The information stored in the brain from past experience.
4. The associations made in the brain between present and past information.

All these factors are, of course, interrelated and interdependent. The physical structure of the brain, for example, is shaped by experience. The degree to which this shaping is possible is limited by the heritage of evolution; regardless of experience, a human brain has a structure which is clearly not the same as a gorilla's brain. Within these evolutionary limits, however, brain structure is modified by its continual interaction with both external and internal environments. Very clear-cut evidence for this is provided by experiments in which cats were raised in total darkness. Under this condition, the visual pathways in the brains did not develop, and a microscopic examination showed that nerve cells in these pathways were dead. Up to a certain age the pathways did retain their capacity to develop, and the animal was able to see when light was restored. After that age, however, the changes in brain structure produced by environment were permanent. In a similar fashion, infant monkeys reared in an abnormal social environment—deprived of their mothers and any other living monkey substitute—grew up to be incurably deviant. A hot water bottle, the sound of a ticking clock, and ample nourishment provided mechanically simply did not offer enough significant environmental stimuli to allow important parts of their emotional brain to mature in a normal fashion.

These experiments are pertinent to the discussion of violence in two ways. First, they indicate that when environmental conditions alter brain structure, the changes may affect behavior because they affect how the brain perceives, *fails* to perceive, or *mis*perceives incoming stimuli. For instance, a person whose violence is related to the presence of brain disease generally does not attack others without what *he* considers to be provocation. What happens is that the brain misperceives some incoming stimulus—a harmless gesture, or a joking remark, let us say—as extremely threatening or enraging, when it is in fact not so. If another driver cuts his car off at a stoplight, his brain interprets it as a deadly insult, and he reacts accordingly. And since his brain may also misinterpret information from his internal environment (that is, his own body—as in the case of depressed blood sugar level) and miscontrol the physical reactions, such as the adrenalin level that accompanies emotion, he will also have great difficulty in governing his rage once it is aroused.

Further, the experiments are pertinent to violence because they show that some stages of brain development apparently occur normally only within certain time limits. If environmental conditions are wrong at the important time, then the resulting anatomical maldevelopment is irreversible, even though the environmental conditions may later be corrected or improved. Once the time had passed for the cats' visual pathways to develop and they had not been stimulated into functioning, it did the animals no good to turn on the light. The point here is that cure, as contrasted with prevention, is not necessarily a matter of eliminating original cause. The kind of violent behavior related to brain malfunction may have its origins in the environment, but once the brain structure has been permanently affected, the violent behavior can no longer be modified by manipulating psychological or social influences. Hoping to rehabilitate such a violent individual through psychotherapy or education, or to improve his character by sending him to jail or by giving him love and understanding—all these methods are irrelevant and will not work. It is the brain malfunction itself that must be dealt with, and only if this fact is recognized is there any chance of changing his behavior.

It is one thing to talk in this abstract way about causal interactions between brain and environment, or of misperceptions of stimuli; it is something else again to see the resulting violent behavior in real life. Take, for example, Paul M., one of our patients—a handsome, muscular 20-year-old who admitted himself to Boston City Hospital because he was afraid he was "going wild" and "didn't want to hurt anybody." Paul came into the hospital after apparently having gone wild in his own apartment. He had ripped plaster off the walls with his bare hands and had smashed a mirror; then, with fragments of broken mirror he had cut deep gashes in his own chest and abdomen.

Let us rather look backward one step from the behavior to the brain processes that produced it. We knew Paul did have some kind of brain damage, at least on a functional level, because he had had an attack of grand mal epilepsy* 5 months earlier following the prolonged ingestion of psychostimulating drugs. Furthermore, he reported that just before his rampage at home, he had suffered a spell of unconsciousness from which he awoke dazed and violent. Paul's brain damage could have been caused by one or more of a number of things we knew about. He had been hit on the head as a child by his brothers and his father, all of whom had violent tempers; and he repeatedly and excessively used alcohol and amphetamines ("speed"), known brain toxins. It is possible, too, that other factors were involved, ones about which we had no evidence—such as infections, abnormal genes, fluctuations in his mother's endocrine level while he was in her womb, or an injury suffered during birth.

Whatever the cause, Paul himself had first noticed the behavioral effects of the damage about the time of his epileptic attack. A very poor boy, one of eight children, he had always been a law breaker with no respect for authority: in the Army he was AWOL twenty times in as many months. He had described himself as "mad at the world," and he consciously modeled his life on the example of an older brother who had been arrested three times for armed robbery and aggravated assault. Despite this admittedly antisocial attitude, Paul did have his own code to which he had always adhered. He might knock someone down, but he would never kill. He might consume large amounts of amphetamines and alcohol, but no LSD; nor did he ever allow himself to get so drunk or so high that he was not able to control his actions. After his grand mal seizure, all this changed. He experienced dreamlike states which convinced him he was losing his mind, and he found he could no longer restrain his violent impulses toward other people or even himself. All of his statements about his changed behavior were verified by his fianceé and acquaintances.

* Epilepsy is described and discussed at length in Chapter 5.

Special x-rays and clinical tests of brain function led to a diagnosis of mild brain damage, and Paul was placed on anti-seizure medication (Dilantin), to which his response has been favorable. He has had no more attacks of rage, and he says he feels once again in control of himself. Paul's case is not unique in that it shows a relationship between brain damage and violent behavior. He is different from other people in his predicament, however, in being helped before he had done much damage to others or to himself.

Paul was fortunate in having a psychiatrist who was able to interpret his symptoms perceptively and who was in an established group of brain clinicians who were willing to see and treat every aspect of his problem. Even today many psychiatric clinics or general hospitals would have dismissed Paul as just another sociopath "on drugs"—or, what is more likely—Paul might have ended up in a prison, where diagnostic and treatment facilities are totally inadequate. Paul is not unusual because he had a single epileptic seizure. This does not mark him as an epileptic and in fact any individual can have a seizure if he is given enough alcohol or drugs and suddenly withdrawn from them. But such an individual has had a sign that his brain is not functioning properly and this sign in Paul plus the evidence of a recent behavior change was enough to spur a full-scale effort to evaluate Paul's brain function. That his function did not fall within the range of normal, or that he required medication does not mean that Paul is now a hopeless cripple. If he refrains from misusing drugs and alcohol, his prognosis is favorable, and perhaps his frightening symptoms were a blessing in disguise for they called attention to the limits of his tolerance. Treatment in Paul's case, of course, must include more than medication. His environment and habit patterns need changing, and fortunately his medication will make him more susceptible to new learning patterns—patterns that can be instilled by intelligent psychotherapy.

Now let us explore the ways in which we perceived that Paul's problem was more than that of a boy with a normal brain, but who was subjected to pernicious environmental influences. Or, more to the point: How we can make a beginning in the hundreds and thousands of violent Pauls all over the country to differentiate those with a normal brain from those with an impaired one, who are in need of medical attention, diagnosis, treatment, and, of course, violence prevention. It is our belief that this beginning can best be made by understanding the organ of behavior—i.e., the brain itself: its function and structure in health and disease; how it produces violence and how it stops it; and how it interacts with its environment. This is a large order because many of the facts about the brain are unknown or just beginning to emerge after years of intensive research. It is our intention then to present the facts we do know in an orderly sequence and tell how these facts are related to violent or attack behavior. Even though many aspects of brain function are unaccounted for, enough information is available to indicate that more brain research is an important key to help unlock the mysteries of human violence.

REFERENCES

Coursin, D. B. "Nutrition and Brain Function." In: *Modern Nutrition in Health and Disease* (M. G. Wohl and R. S. Goodhart, eds.). Philadelphia, Lea & Febiger, 1968.

Eisenberg, L. "Normal Child Development." In: *Comprehensive Textbook of Psychiatry* (A. Freedman and H. Kaplan, eds.). Baltimore, Williams & Wilkins Co., 1967.

Eisenhower, M. E. (Chairman), *et al.* To Establish Justice, To Insure Domestic Tranquility: Final Report of the National Commission on the Causes and Prevention of Violence. Washington, D.C., U. S. Government Printing Office, 1969.

Ervin, F. R. and Lion, J. R. Clinical evaluation of the violent patient. National Commission for the Causes and Prevention of Violence. March, 1969. (In press)

Facts on the Major Killing and Crippling Diseases in the United States Today. New York, The National Health Education Committee, Inc., 1966.

Harlow, H. F. "The Development of Affectional Patterns in Infant Monkeys." In: *Determinants of Infant Behavior* (B. M. Foss, ed.). London, Methuen, 1961, pp. 75–88.

Harlow, H. F. "Development of the Second and Third Affectional Systems in Macaque Monkeys." In: *Research Approaches to Psychiatric Problems: A Symposium* (T. T. Tourlentes, S. L. Pollock, and H. E. Himwich, eds.), New York, Grune & Stratton, 1962, pp. 209–229.

Harlow, H. F. The heterosexual affectional system in monkeys. *Amer. Psychol. 17*:1–9, 1962.

Helfer, R. E., and Kempe, C. H. (eds.) *The Battered Child.* Chicago, The University of Chicago Press, 1968.

Hubel, D. H. Effects of distortion of sensory imput on the visual system of kittens. *The Physiologist 10:*17–45, 1967.

Kihlberg, J. "Head Injury in Automobile Accidents," In: *Head Injury: Conference Proceedings.* (W. F. Caveness and A. E. Walker, eds.). Philadelphia, Lippincott, 1966.

Lion, J. R., Bach-y-Rita, G., and Ervin, F. R. Enigmas of violence. *Science 164:*1465, 1969.

Masland, R. Testimony before subcommittee of the committee on appropriations, House of Representatives, 89th Congress, first session, part 3. Cited by: Laufer, M. W. "Brain Disorders." In: *Comprehensive Textbook of Psychiatry* (A. Freedman and H. Kaplan, eds.). Baltimore, Williams & Wilkins Co., 1967.

World Almanac, 1970.

Appendix

Brain Dysfunction: Some Thoughts on the Magnitude of the Problem

We use the terminology of brain dysfunction as outlined by Denhoff and Robinault. These workers etiologically classify dysfunction into cerebral palsy, mental retardation, convulsive disorders, and hyperkinetic-behavior disorders.

Statistical estimates of the prevalence of these diseases in the United States (National Health Education Committee Publication) are as follows: Cerebral palsy, half a million. Mental retardation, six million, Convulsive disorders, two million. Hyperkinetic-behavior disorders, 5–10 per cent of school population (Masland), which is approximately two-and-a-half million.

War injuries and accidents represent two major sources of brain injury. With regard to the former, no figures are available to indicate what general combined percentages of the total of 1.5 million men wounded in the past three major and present Vietnam war have sustained head injury. Figures do exist for automobile accidents; head injury is the most frequent lethal injury in such accidents. Estimates are that three million persons sustain injuries in motor vehicle mishaps each year. In 33 per cent of head injuries, internal tissue and organs of the head are injured (Kihlberg). Statistics indicating the clinical sequellae of accidents are not available.

We draw attention to an increasing literature showing the detrimental effects of maternal and social deprivation (Eisenberg) as well as protein malnutrition (Coursin) upon developing human intelligence and other aspects of perception and cognition. The reservoir of potential "casualties" here would appear to be high.

Chapter 2

Our Emotional Brain

Not in utter nakedness,
But trailing clouds of glory do we come,
From God who is our home.

That is the poet's vision. It may be true, but there are others who think that what we trail from our past are snaky skeins of degrading animal instincts and bestial impulses drawn from the primordial slime out of which we emerged.

So far as we can judge from the scientific evidence, neither of these partial statements is adequate. Human nature unquestionably had an animal origin and it is still animal nature. But animal nature is not degraded nature. It has dignity and worth and it increases in competence to order self and environment as we pass from lower to higher forms.

C. S. Herrick

The Evolution of Human Nature

Although some biologists, including Konrad Lorenz, believe that individual violence against others of the same species is a distinctively and distressingly human form of activity, even they do not deny that the brain machinery directing this behavior in man is part of the biological heritage he shares with his fellow vertebrates. And, to some degree, so is the violent behavior itself, for it is basically akin to that exhibited by all other animals in threatening situations.

Any animal, regardless of its species, reacts to a life-threatening attack with one of two patterns of behavior: either with flight, or with aggression and violence—that is, fight. The brain always acts as a unit in directing any behavior; consequently, the mechanisms in the brain that initiate and limit these two dissimilar patterns of self-preservation are closely linked to one another, as well as to all other parts of the brain; and their proper functioning depends on the sychronization of many complex and delicately balanced subsystems. Because self-preservation is so often associated with violence, it is easy to see that a disturbance or disorder of brain mechanisms has the potential of releasing violent behavior, even when the circumstances do not call for it. Moreover, the chance of such a disturbance or disorder occurring increases with any increase in the complexity of the nervous system, and also with any increase in the variety of environmental stimuli to which an animal must respond in order to survive.

Violent behavior as one aspect of self-preservation has existed on this earth for hundreds of millions of years. It is not surprising, therefore, to find that the mechanisms that *initiate* it are in the deepest, most primitive center of the vertebrate brain—the brain stem.* Nor is it surprising to find that mechanisms for *controlling* violence and other brain stem functions are situated in the deepest and oldest part of the vertebrate "large brain" or cerebrum. This oldest part of the cerebrum is called the *limbic system* or *limbic brain.* The limbic brain developed about 400 million years ago and flourished 150 million years ago, when reptiles still dominated the earth's crust; and its structures and functions were modified, regulated, and influenced by the "new brain" or "neocortex" that appeared

* The brain stem is the tube of nervous tissue that connects the large brain to the spinal cord and houses the mechanisms that control breathing, heart beat, and sleep or wakefulness.

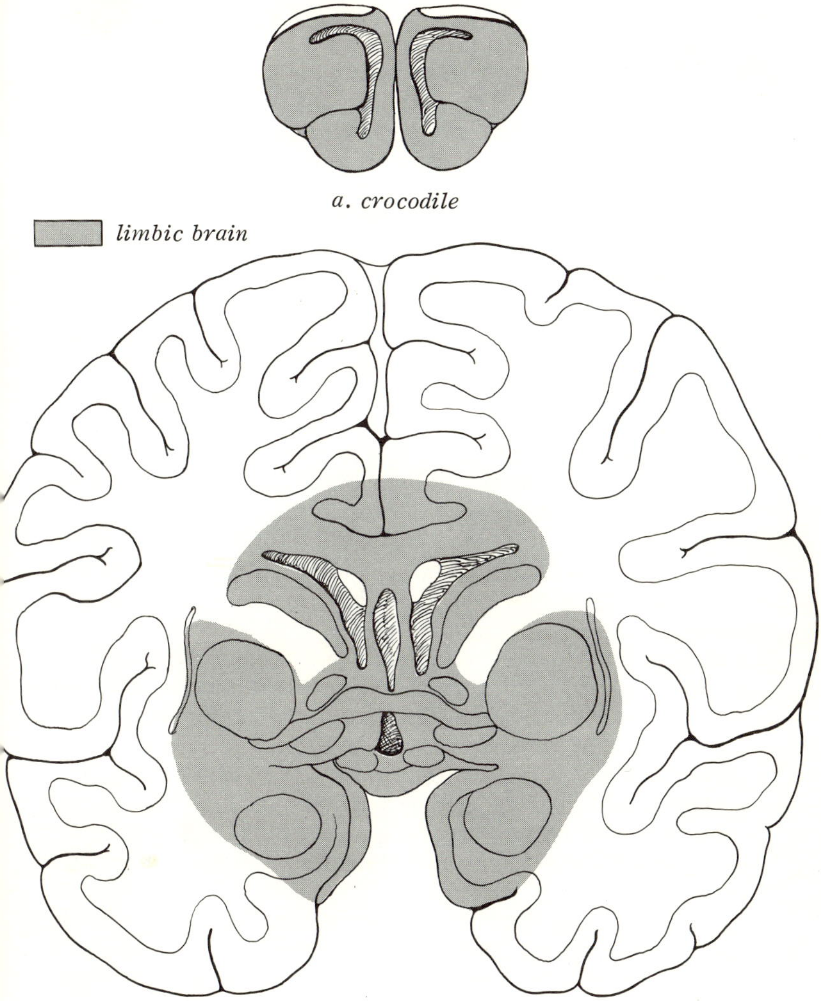

FIG. 1. A schematic cross section of (*a*) crocodile brain (*b*) human brain. Coronal (cross) section of human cerebrum is contrasted with section from crocodile's brain. Limbic portion of both brains darkened by overlay. Crocodile's cerebrum or large brain consists almost entirely of limbic brain, while markedly greater-sized human brain is accounted for by development of neocortex or "new brain."

ages later in animals such as the human. The limbic system is also called the "nose" brain because one of its oldest functions is to detect and interpret odors; smelling and interpreting odors are hence closely associated in all animals with the "emergency responses" to a threatening environment.

The limbic part of the brain in amphibians and reptiles and even mammals governs many kinds of behavior besides violence. After all, primitive reptile brains such as the crocodile's, which consists mostly of limbic brain, may be relatively simple in comparison to the brain of a chimpanzee or man, but it has nonetheless been adequate for the crocodile* to have survived for millions of years. A schematic cross section of the crocodile's brain (Fig. 1) shows that the old or limbic brain makes up most of the brain mass, and that there is very little nonlimbic cortex.

A cross section of the human brain (Fig. 1) shows a much greater proportion of neocortex to old brain. The overall size of the brain has increased tremendously (about tenfold), and this increase is accounted for almost entirely by neocortical tissue. Evolution has pushed the limbic brain toward the center and into close proximity with the brain stem—that is, the structure that directly initiates fight-or-flight behavior. In man, the limbic brain influences and regulates functions of the brain stem but is in turn influenced by the more complex integrating mechanisms of the neocortex (Fig. 1). Violence is thus still part of man's vast repertoire of potential behavior; however, the neocortex and its associated systems have elaborated the ancient simplicities of fight or flight into patterns of destruction far more colorful and controlled than those of any other animal species.

Basically, then, violent behavior is governed most closely by the structures of the limbic brain. In order to get a clear picture of these structures, let us begin with a short discussion of the central nervous system and how it evolved. In primitive vertebrates (and in the human embryo, whose development

* We are referring in this volume to the order, not the species.

FIG. 2. Prenatal stages in development of human brain. Embryonic development of human brain is depicted in six diagrams. Darkened portions of each figure represent limbic brain and stippled areas the neocortex or new brain. Growth of the new brain is more rapid than the limbic brain, which is finally surrounded by new brain structures.

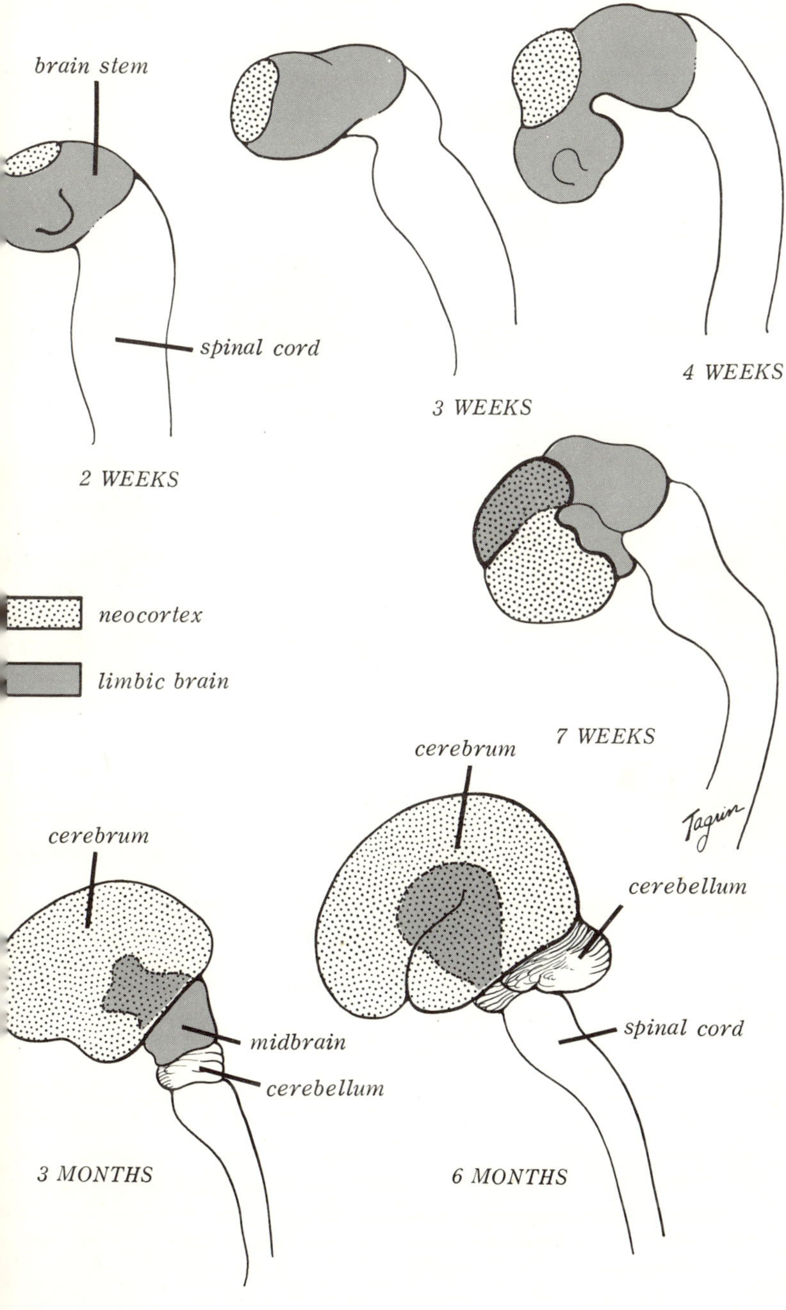
brain stem
spinal cord
2 WEEKS
3 WEEKS
4 WEEKS
7 WEEKS
neocortex
limbic brain
cerebrum
midbrain
cerebellum
3 MONTHS
cerebrum
cerebellum
spinal cord
6 MONTHS

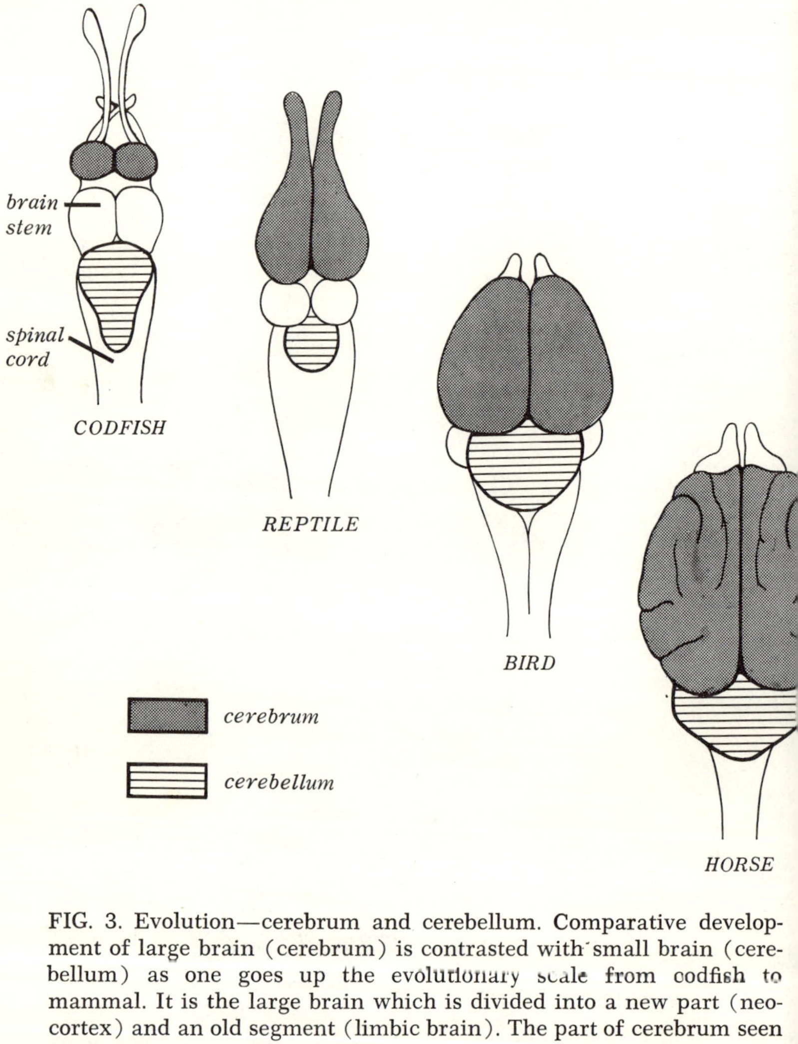

FIG. 3. Evolution—cerebrum and cerebellum. Comparative development of large brain (cerebrum) is contrasted with small brain (cerebellum) as one goes up the evolutionary scale from codfish to mammal. It is the large brain which is divided into a new part (neocortex) and an old segment (limbic brain). The part of cerebrum seen from above is mostly neocortex in mammals.

recapitulates phylogenetic history,*) the brain started as a tube of delicate nervous tissue extending the entire length of the organism, protected by the individual bones of the spine and the cranium (Fig. 2). That part of the tube which was covered

*The human embryo in its development goes through stages roughly resembling lower animal forms—e.g., fish, amphibian, reptiles, and then mammals.

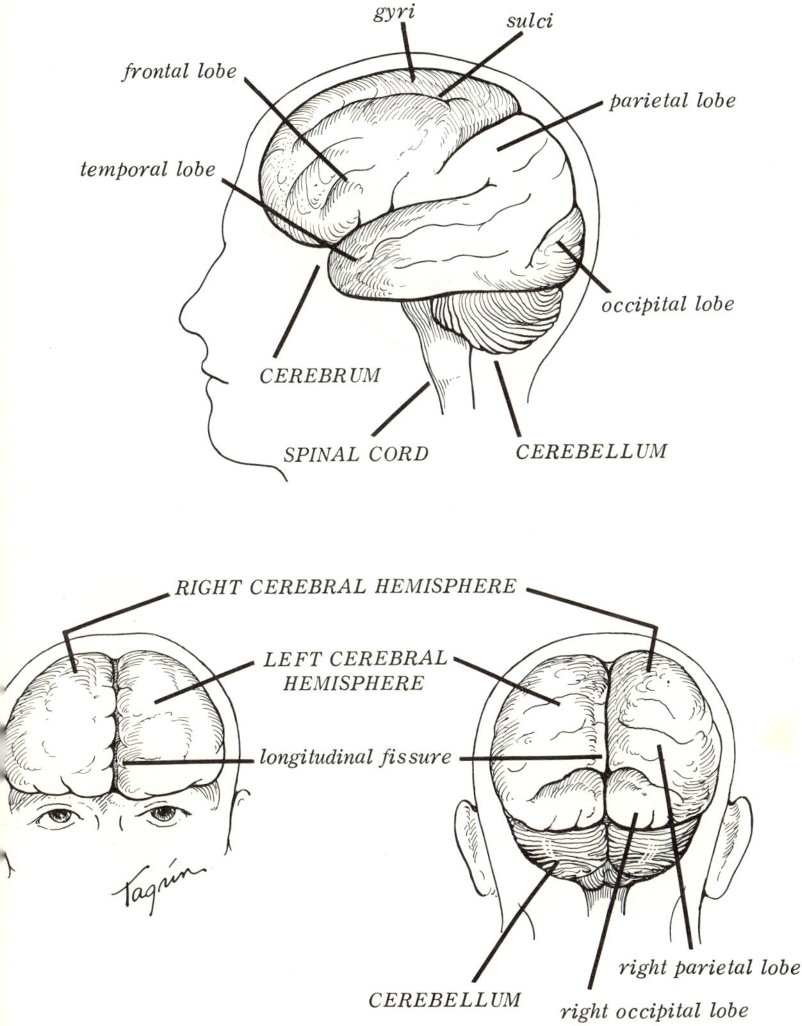

FIG. 4. Outline of adult head, showing brain in lateral, anterior, and posterior views. Surface landmarks of the brain are depicted in side front and rear views of the head.

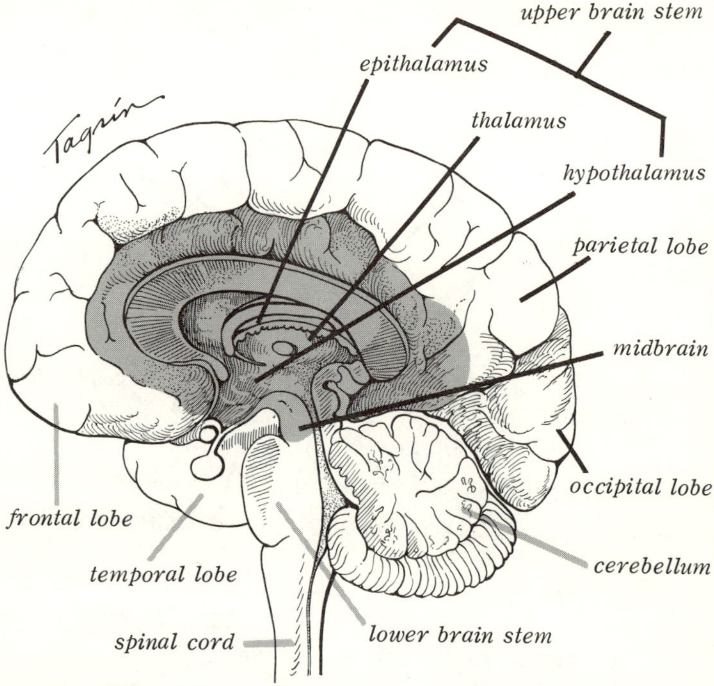

FIG. 5. Medial surface of right cerebral hemisphere and brain stem. Limbic areas of brain are shaded in this sagittal section of *midline* structures which is prepared by separating the two hemispheres and dividing the brain stem lengthwise into two equal parts.

by the backbone evolved into the spinal cord; the upper end of the tube—the head ganglion—which was covered by the cranium evolved into the brain stem.

During the course of evolution, two paired bubbles of brain tissues expanded out of the brain stem (Fig. 3). The lower pair emerged from the lower brain stem and formed the cerebellum. The cerebellum controls the sense of balance, and integrates the muscles used in vertebrate movement—walking, swimming, flying, and running

The upper pair of bubbles, which together are called the cerebrum or large brain, emerged from either side of the uppermost portion of the brain stem. The dividing line between them is marked by a large longitudinal fissure. Each half of the cerebrum is itself divided into lobes, named according to their position: the frontal lobe is in the front part of the skull;

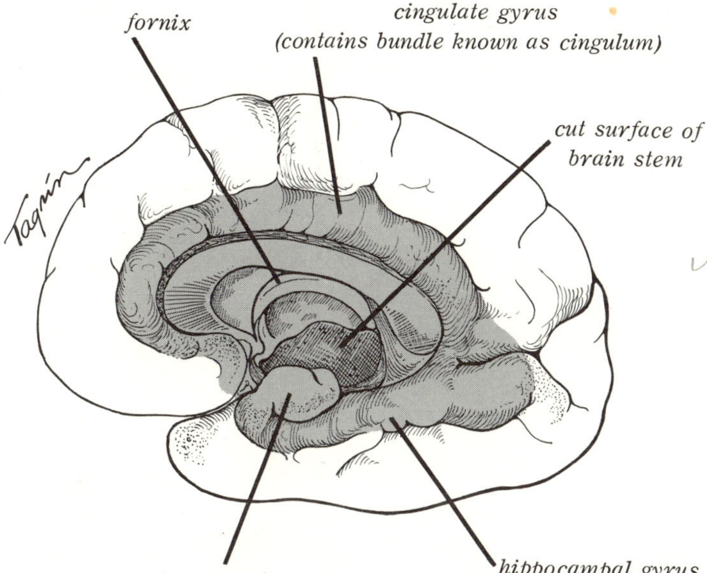

FIG. 6. Medial surface of right cerebral hemisphere (lower brain stem removed). This is another midline view of the brain, but the brain stem has been removed to give a clear view of inner surface of entire cerebral hemisphere, including inner (medial) portion of temporal lobe. Shaded areas are part of limbic system.

the occipital lobe is in the back (under the occipital bone, which forms the back of the skull); the parietal lobe is on the top of the brain (under the bones that form the roof of the skull); and the temporal lobe lies just beneath the temple and ear (Fig. 4).

The structures comprising the limbic brain are today generally considered to include the upper part of the brain stem, as well as the deep structures of the cerebrum (Fig. 5.). These limbic structures still bear the names given to them by ancient Greek anatomists. They called the upper brain stem "the thalamus," which means an inner "bridal chamber," for it is the place where the senses—touch, vision, and hearing—can be joined. The roof of this chamber is thus the *epi*thalamus and the floor the *hypo*thalamus. The limbic brain itself (Fig. 6) takes its name from "limbus" the Latin word for "border," since it prominently outlines the inner surface of each cerebral hemi-

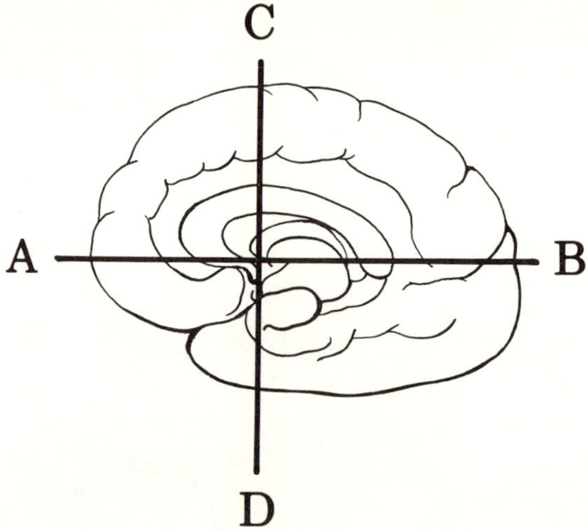
C
A
B
D

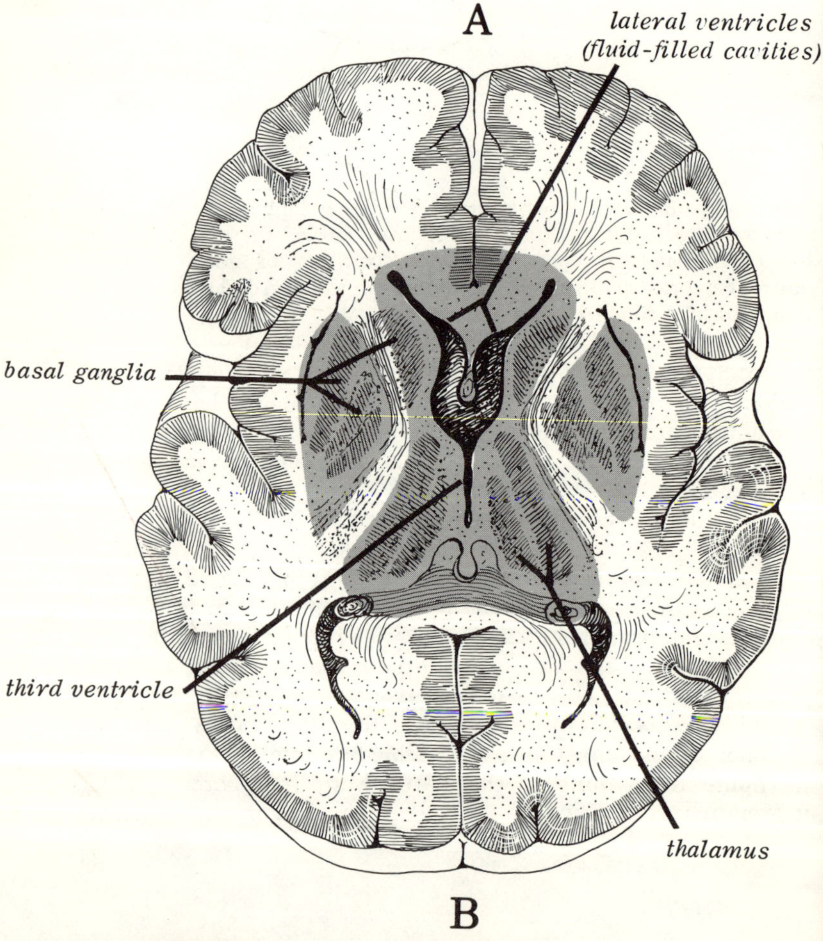
A
lateral ventricles
(fluid-filled cavities)
basal ganglia
third ventricle
thalamus
B

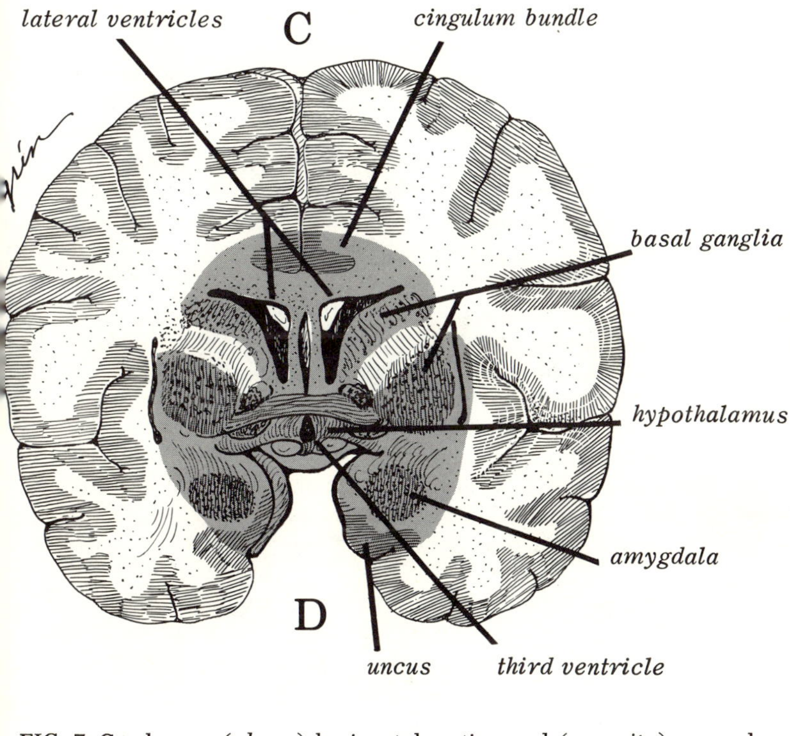

FIG. 7. Cerebrum: (*above*) horizontal section and (*opposite*) coronal section. Horizontal (*A–B*) and coronal (*C–D*) section of brain hemispheres allows us to inspect some details of deeper limbic brain structures. These limbic areas are shaded in the diagrams.

sphere. This border is C-shaped. The top of the C is called the cingulum—the Latin word for "girdle" or "belt." The bottom of the C is called the hippocampus because it curls upon itself and looks, when viewed in a longitudinal section, like a "seahorse," which is what hippocampus means.

Other parts of the brain associated with the functions of the limbic brain include cell-packed areas deep in the cerebrum: among these are the basal ganglia; the septal nuclei, which include groups of cells near the inner wall, or septum of the fluid-filled cavities of the brain; the undersurface of the frontal lobe; the midbrain, which is comprised of the middle portion of the brain stem; and finally, the amygdala—meaning "almond" —an almond-shaped nucleus in the front of the temporal lobe (Fig. 7). These structures were not part of the limbic lobe of the older anatomists, but they have been included in the limbic system as delineated by modern brain physiologists.

The amygdala is a particularly important structure, with extensive connections to many portions of the limbic system. Its connections to the hypothalamus are especially large, and it exerts an important modulating influence over emotional activity. It is well to remember, however, that the amygdala is simply not one large structure with a single function. Anatomists have been able to define from 9 to 14 different anatomical areas within this nucleus, each of which may have a separate function. Despite this complexity, alterations in the structure or function of an animal's amygdala invariably produce changes in its behavior state, with results ranging from placidity to terrifying rage.

To sum up: when we refer to the "emotional brain," the "limbic brain," or the "limbic system," we shall mean the cingulum, the hippocampus, the thalamic and hypothalamic nuclei, and the more complex masses of the basal ganglia, midbrain, and amygdala. (Fig. 7.). This system has a wide range of functions including the modulation and control of fight-or-flight behavior. In the next chapters, we shall see how this constellation of anatomical structures is related to emotional behavior, especially violent behavior; and further, how brain disease can disrupt its ability to control behavior.

REFERENCES

Arey, L. B. *Developmental Anatomy.* Philadelphia, Saunders, 1926.

Crosby, E. C., Humphrey, T., and Lauer, E. W. *Correlated Anatomy of the Nervous System.* New York, MacMillan, 1962.

Delmas, A., and Pertuiset, B. La topométirc encéphalique chez l'homme (noyau rouge, centre median, noyau amygdalien). *Presse Méd., 82:*1784–1787, 1952.

Herrick C. J. *The Evolution of Human Nature.* Austin, Univer. Texas Press, 1956.

Kaada, B. R. "Cingulate, Posterior Orbital, Anterior Insular and Temporal Pole Cortex." In *Handbook of Physiology, Sec. 1., Neurophysiology, Vol. II* (John Field, ed.-in-chief). Washington, D. C., American Physiology Society, 1960, pp. 1345–1372.

McLardy, T. "Some Cell and Fibre Peculiarities of Uncal Hippocampus." In *The Rhinencephalon and Related Structures: Progress in Brain Research, Vol. 3* (W. Bargmann and J. P. Schade, eds.). New York, Elsevier, 1963, pp. 71–88.

Papez, J. W. *Comparative Neurology.* New York, Hafner, 1929.

Pernkopf, E. *Atlas of Topographical and Applied Human Anatomy, Vol. I.: Head and Neck.* Philadelphia, Saunders, 1963.

Singer, M., and Yakovlev, P. I. *The Human Brain in Sagittal Section.* Springfield, Ill., Thomas, 1964.

Spalteholz, W. *Hand-Atlas of Human Anatomy, Vol. III; Viscera, Brain, Nerves, Sense-Organs* (2nd ed., in English). Philadelphia, Lippincott, 1846.

Spiegel, E. A., and Wycis, H. T. *Stereoencephalotomy (Thalamotomy and Related Procedures): Part I. Methods and Stereotaxis Atlas of the Human Brain.* New York, Grune & Stratton, 1952.

Talairach, J., David, M., Tournoux, P., Corredor, H., and Kvasina, T. *Atlas d'Anatomie Stereotaxique.* Paris, Masson, 1957.

Villiger, E. *Brain and Spinal Cord.* Philadelphia, Lippincott, 1912.

Williams, D. Man's temporal lobe. *Brain 91* (pt. 4):639–654, 1968.

Chapter 3

Rage, Anger, and Fear

> ***Fear, rage, and pain, and the pangs of hunger are all primitive experiences which human beings share with the lower animals. These experiences are properly classed as among the most powerful that determine the action of men and beast. A knowledge of the conditions which attend these experiences, therefore, is of general and fundamental importance in the interpretation of behavior.***
>
> ***Walter B. Cannon***
>
> **Bodily Changes in Pain, Hunger, Fear, and Rage**

In the last chapter, we defined the brain structures that are involved in the control and initiation of violent behavior. It is not enough to know what these structures are, however; we must also determine how they function—which areas govern aggressive behavior, which areas limit attack, which areas initiate and which stop violence. Three kinds of experimental procedures are used to relate brain function to behavior of any kind, all of which have been utilized in attempts to define the function of the limbic system in the complex brain of higher animals. These procedures include: (1) recording changes in electrical activity in the brain; (2) removing part of the brain, a procedure called ablation; and (3) stimulating areas of the brain with chemicals or a weak electric current.

Recording

Since brain activity is accompanied by electrical signals, it is possible to measure changes in this neuroelectric activity during different behavioral states by applying wires (electrodes) to the brain surface, to points within the brain, or to the surface of the head. When signals from these wires are amplified, they can be recorded as voltage-versus-time curves on a writing instrument such as a brain wave machine, or displayed visibly on the fluorescent screen of a cathode ray oscilloscope. It is assumed that if the patterns of these curves change consistently during the experiment when there are observed behavioral responses to the changing experimental conditions, then the two phenomena—i.e., electrical and behavioral—are related. And, of course, this relationship can be confirmed experimentally by the application of statistical techniques.

Most of the recording studies made on violent behavior have been made on humans, rather than on the usual lab animals such as cats or monkeys. However, a few studies on animals designed to investigate mechanisms of learning indicate that the amygdala and the hippocampus are particularly responsive to changes in the environment. For example, the arrival of a strange animal, including a new human experimenter, initiates a flurry of electrical activity in these brain structures, which disappears as soon as the animal gets used to the stranger. This electrical activity coincides in time with searching or orienting movements that prepare the animal for flight or fight: the eyes and ears are focused on the unfamiliar; the animal sniffs and adopts an alert posture; and its heart rate, blood pressure, and respiration increase. Whether there is a detectable change of electrical activity during any final act of attack or retreat has not been experimentally determined. In animals with normal brains, the limited evidence available would suggest that there is not a unique change.

Ablation

The surgical removal or ablation of part of the brain makes it possible to study how the remaining brain structures function. The interpretation of ablation data is not an easy matter. For one thing, brain structures are related to one another in complex ways; for another, each half of the cerebrum has great reserves of functional capacity. Indeed, some people who have had as much as half their brains removed because of brain cysts dating back to the time of their birth show little or no loss of those so-called higher functions most people ordinarily associate with the brain—such as intelligence, memory, or capacity to plan.

One of the ablation experiments used in studying violent behavior was done on cats; it involved removing all neocortex (a procedure called decortication). This left behind as functioning brain only the limbic system and other deep structures such as the brain stem. Such a "limbic animal" shows no change in its basic "personality." Friendly, gentle animals continue to purr and be affectionate after decortication; more aggressive, intractable animals remain difficult to handle. All these cats, however, were quick to respond to threatening or painful stimuli with explosive emotionality. Tail-pinching, having air blown in their faces, the appearance of a competitive male—situations which might make any cat "angry"—made the decorticated animals attack with the kind of ferocity that seems possible only when the limbic brain has been freed from neocortical control.

A series of ablation experiments have shown what happens when small areas of the limbic brain are removed. This sort of experiment began to attract attention more than 20 years ago when Heinrich Klüver and Paul Bucy removed both temporal lobes in a rhesus monkey. Taking out the temporal lobes deprives the monkey of its amygdala, hippocampus, hippocampal gyrus, and piriform cortex, all structures of the limbic system; in addition, the temporal neocortex is lost as well. Normally, unless they are carefully handled and trained, rhesus monkeys will attack when a man approaches them. However, after both temporal lobes have been removed, they are placid, can be easily handled, and do not respond aggressively even to attack by other, normal monkeys within the social group. Moreover, they become seriously disturbed in other ways: they are oversexed and mount other animals or inanimate objects indiscriminately, and they not only eat more than a normal amount but tend to put every new object into their mouths, including objects that ordinarily provoke fear, such as small snakes. The results of a number of similar operations on other kinds of animals over the last two decades indicate that the taming effect discovered by Klüver and Bucy is specifically related to amygdala destruction. Localized removal of the amygdala will tame a predatory and vicious lynx or a wolverine. A special and well-studied strain of killer rats no longer attack mice after their amygdalas are taken out; and animals that are traditionally fearful of men, like the mallard duck, can be captured by hand after surgical damage to the amygdaloid region. Occasionally in cats, a paradoxical response is noted and amygdala removal will make a placid animal vicious.

A particularly dramatic demonstration of the effect of amygdalectomy was provided when an experimenter named Jack Downer surgically separated the two halves of a rhesus monkey's brain so that its right eye projected visual images only to the right hemisphere. Downer then removed the monkey's right amygdala but not the left, after which the animal exhibited a truly split personality. When approached from the right, it was a docile animal. When approached from the left, however, it reacted with the combination of fearful and aggressive behavior that is normal for rhesus monkeys.

In contrast to this taming effect of removing the amygdala, other experiments have shown that destroying small areas of the ventromedial nucleus of the hypothalamus in cats and rats produces a permanently ferocious animal, difficult to handle. The results of these experiments, as well as the fact that there are many fiber connections between the hypothalamic nucleus and the amygdala, seem to imply that the amygdala may be controlled through this nucleus, since its removal leads to persistent amygdala excitement, indicated by the readiness for attack. Removal of the aymgdala, in turn, prevents the display of attack behavior in spite of normal provocation. Indeed, neurosurgeons have surgically removed areas of the amygdala to treat assaultive behavior in patients for whom this symptom was a disabling feature of some other brain disease.

Stimulation

There is another way to relate brain structure to behavior, and that is by stimulating the brain through wires implanted by the stereotactic technique.* A surgical team inserts tiny wires

* Stereotactic surgery is described in detail in Chapter 6.

(electrodes) or tubes containing chemicals into a specific brain structure. Then they pass a weak electrical current through the wire or release a minute quantity of the chemical within the tube. The effect is to excite activity in that part of the brain. While this kind of stimulation is artificial in the sense that normal electrical or chemical brain signals are not duplicated, it does seem to represent a crude approximation of normal functioning as judged from the resulting behavior. To the person or animal whose brain is being examined, stimulation of the visual system gives rise to the sensation of a formless flash of light. If the stimulation affects the auditory system, he experiences a buzzing sound. Stimulating the surface area of his brain that controls arm movement produces movement in the hand or arm, although the precise movement depends not only on the point on the brain that is stimulated but also on the arm's position and the total posture.

Stimulation offers perhaps the best way to get a clear idea of the way the limbic system works. Stimulation throughout a wide area in the limbic brain of an awake and freely moving cat with implanted electrodes turns the animal into a Halloween cat—its back arches, it growls and spits, its hair bristles, and its pupils widen. Whether the stimulation makes it attack or flee depends largely on environmental circumstances. It may try to get away from its surroundings, but if there is a suitable object available, it will usually launch an attack. Cats so stimulated have attacked rats, other cats, large dogs, teddy bears, and experimenters.

Cats stimulated in this way will learn to seek objects to attack. Furthermore, they are motivated to attack an object whether it be a mouse or another cat, and to do so they will run mazes, open doors, and climb barriers. They thus behave as if the aggressive act induced by limbic stimulation were "rewarding"—like food or water. This is not simply the stimulation of an "on" point in the brain, which produces an immediate response like switching on an electric light. It is instead the turning on of *motivation* or *reward-seeking* behavior, and in this case the reward is the aggressive act.

Several areas of the limbic brain will elicit this kind of attack behavior under electrical stimulation. These areas include the amygdala, the middle of the hypothalamus, the connections between them, and the portion of the midbrain to which the hypothalamus is connected. If this part of the midbrain is blocked or inactivated by electric currents, or by lowering the temperature in that part of the brain, the attack produced by stimulation is temporarily blocked. If this inactivation is lifted, the animal will usually flee rather than attack in response to the same stimulation.

If the side of the hypothalamus rather than the middle is stimulated, the cat behaves somewhat differently. It meows and spits less, its hair does not bristle so much, and its aggressive reactions—slinking, seizing objects in its mouth, pawing in holes, and pouncing—are closer to hunting behavior than to defensive behavior. Certain kinds of lesions in the midbrain also produce this type of hunting behavior, to the degree that the animal spends its entire waking life slinking, seizing, pawing in holes, and pouncing.

Another significant finding from these studies of experimentally produced attack behavior is that simultaneous electrical stimulation in other parts of the brain will stop the attack. Many of these "stop points" are within the limbic system, and some are points which are apparently rewarding, judging by results of other experiments in which so-called self-stimulation was used. In the attack situation, it is not that stimulation of this "reward" system will stop all performance, but rather that the animal no longer seems angry or fearful; he will respond to other things around him; he will eat or groom. As we shall describe in Chapter 7, the subjective reports of men similarly stimulated confirm this interpretation. Indeed, the existence of this parallel system of tranquility is the key to an understanding of the systems that control attack behavior; this phenomenon has great potential significance for the practical treatment of violent behavior in man.

Conclusions

To summarize: the results of the experiments cited above on recording, ablating, and stimulating animal brains seem to indicate clearly that there is a definable neural system which organizes effective and directed attack behavior, and that this system is linked to structures of the limbic brain. The system can be activated by events within the environment, or by artificial stimulation of the limbic brain; and removal or destruction of specific limbic structures leads to predictable behavioral changes especially in regard to the display of fight or flight reactions.

Interpretation of the experimental data in this chapter poses an interesting philosophical problem. It seems clear that there exists within the brain a definable neural system which organizes effective and directed attack behavior. This system has a long and honorable evolutionary past; indeed, it was necessary for survival and still exists in mammals of normally peaceful mien.

As this chapter indicates, the existence of this neural system is easy to demonstrate. One common response to this demonstration is that such a mechanism implies an aggressive instinct, an inborn, inescapable drive to kill; and people divide promptly into two customary groups in applying these findings to man. One, insisting that man is potentially not evil, denies the applicability of these brain mechanisms to behavior. The other agrees gloomily that "that's human nature" and calls for more repressive force to keep it in line. With these familiar responses dominating much of the recent public discussions on aggression and violence, it is worth trying to be *very* clear about our interpretation of these data.

That the machinery for attack behavior exists is quite clear. The evidence cited demonstrates that it is not identical to (although it overlaps the brain mechanisms necessary for) effective predatory activity in those animals which live by hunting. That is, it is present for self-defense, as a response to perceived threat, and, in general, is as ready to authorize flight as attack. Thus the limbic brain cannot be thought of solely as an aggression system.

It is also important to emphasize that in the normal human brain, the fight or flight response is just one of many in the human behavioral repertoire under the control of the "new" brain. The limbic system is called on to contribute to a wide spectrum of human and other mammalian actions and feelings, but it need never be used at full power. After all, keeping matches in the home does not imply that the home-owner is a pyromaniac. The machinery for arson is present; and, in fact, the matches may be used with some emotional pleasure on fireplace logs. In well-ordered hands, however, there is no danger that these matches will be used for arson.

Similarly, in the well-ordered brain, the mechanisms of violence are there, but they need never be out of control. If they are, one of two things has occurred: either the limbic system has become pathologically hyperactive due to a lesion or stimulation, or its neocortical (control) inputs have become abnormal. These inputs are heavily dependent on learning, the process which determines the microstructure of the brain after birth and which incorporates the past (including cultural and family patterns of behavior) into the brain. Therefore, a brain programmed in a particular way by a particular culture might well perceive threats more intensively or more frequently than another, and hence call the limbic organization into action for violent attack. The understanding of distortions in brain learning, which may pervade an entire culture, are properly the concern of psychologists, sociologists, anthropologists, and other social scientists. At present we have only tentative clues as to the impact of experience on brain structure and organization. Indeed it may turn out to be most useful, from the standpoint of preventing violent behavior, to modify the environment before brain structure is "set" too solidly, because afterwards even the most drastic environmental manipulation may be ineffective.

Ethology

Another method of studying brain function—including attack behavior—is to look at the behavior of a whole animal as it interacts with its usual environment. These kinds of studies have been carried on a number of animal species, including man. Unfortunately, almost all of the investigators of violent behavior carry over a particular philosophical or ethical opinion to the interpretation of their work. For example, the question as to whether man is intrinsically violent has been answered in the affirmative by a number of distinguished students of behavior. In the first half of this century, William James and Sigmund Freud made the most explicit and notable formulations of this view, and did so when mankind was on the eve of the two World Wars—behaving with a minimum of rational judgment. It is sobering to reflect that this argument has again become intellectually prominent in the past five years, this time supported by data from observations of animals in a natural habitat. These "ethological" studies, attempting to define the fixed patterns of behavior of animals in their social and ecological interactions, have become increasingly important to behavioral science in the last two decades. Konrad Lorenz is the godfather of, and the most prominent spokesman for, this field of ethology, even though he is not universally agreed with.* His published observations on the aggressive behavior

* A thorough critique of Konrad Lorenz (*On Aggression*) and Robert Ardrey (the *Territorial Imperative*) is contained in a volume entitled *Man and Aggression,* edited by M. F. Ashley Montagu. The most telling arguments against the validity of Lorenz's judgement of human behavior is contained in the chapter written by Zuckerman. Unfortunately other parts of this volume are marred by the prejudices of some of its authors. For example, Montagu has dug up the old nature-vs.-nurture controversy. And on page 11 he states: "The fact is, that with the exception of the instinctoid reactions in infants to sudden withdrawals of support and to sudden loud noises, the human being is entirely instinctless."

How does Montagu explain the suckling of the breast by a newborn human infant? This is not a learned response and it is just one of many behavior patterns present in the newborn which are necessary for survival. Montagu has overstated his case and weakened his argument. This is too bad because his conclusions regarding the lack of innate violence in human beings are quite sensible.

Again, on page 53, J. P. Scott suggests that Lorenz's idea, "aggression is an instinct," is not valid. He bases his criticism on the fact that aggressive responses usually require an external initiating stimulus. But here again if we examine the suckling response in human infants we note that it often has to be evoked by cutaneous stimulation of the infant's lips. But once this stimulation has evoked the response, that response continues in a rhythmic fashion for 30 to 50 seconds without further initiating stimulation. Just because suckling requires a cutaneous stimulus does not mean that it is not a complex automatic behavioral pattern which can be defined as instinct; Scott's criticism of Lorenz on this score is not valid.

Ironically both Montagu and Lorenz are guilty of oversimplifying the mechanisms of human behavior. All basic neurological mechanisms, including respiration, are subject to profound modification by learning. For example, a patient with hyperventilation syndrome has not suddenly developed a breathing mechanism that is entirely learned, even though his breathing pattern has been modified by learning. A man who requires a sexual partner in a black nightgown for sexual arousal may have modified his copulatory behavior by learning, but his pelvic thrust during orgasm is still a reflection of the basic organization of his central nervous system—an organization that he not only shares with all other human males but also with most mammals. In a similar fashion, the human *fight*-or-*flight* of fish, birds, and mammals are included in his monograph, *On Aggression,* in which he emphasizes the stereotyped, ritualistic, and usually harmless modes of aggression that result, for example, between two male animals vying for a female, or that occur when the territory of one animal or group is invaded by another animal or group of the same species. He has demonstrated the interaction of other behavioral drives in modulating aggressive behavior to prevent physical violence within the species.

On the other hand, serious intraspecific aggression does occur when one community of social insects (bees, termites, and ants) is mixed with another community of the same insects. A massacre will ensue if the human experimenter inhumanely tries to mix two colonies. Large families of rodents also behave in a similar fashion. Both the brown rat and the house mouse get along very peaceably with their own clans or families; but if a strange rodent of the same species is put into their nest, they will literally tear it apart. This fate may even befall a member of a rat family unlucky enough to lose the characteristic odor of the clan. It is interesting to note that here again odor is the stimulus which sets off aggressive attack in members of the same species and, as we have seen, the sense of smell is intimately connected with the limbic brain.

The vicious, intraspecific attack manifested by the rat families stands in marked contrast to the intraspecific behavior of well-armed predators such as the wolf and lion. It is the contention of several investigators that these animal species living in moderate or large social groups have unusually good control mechanisms to prevent serious intraspecies violence, even though ritual battle for mates and social dominance does occur. If these controls did not exist, it would be difficult for such a species to survive.

This is also true of primate behavior, as indicated by field studies of apes and monkeys reported recently in a volume edited by Devore. Far from being intensely violent (an opinion we often reach when trying to handle monkeys in the laboratory), most

response can be modified into a violent pattern by learning, but this does not mean that the basic mechanism for fight or flight is not represented by neural arrangements in the hypothalamus. Moreover, it is our opinion that violent patterns occur more frequently when these basic mechanisms are deranged by disease or injury.

species of monkeys and apes exhibit little intraspecies violence. Their attack behavior, particularly within the same group, is usually short-lived and extremely limited in scope. Most conflicts, in fact, are settled by symbolic displays and rituals. This is true even of the mountain gorilla, whose prodigious strength would make him a formidable opponent. These large animals are apparently docile vegetarians and are unlikely to attack man unless they are cornered or severely threatened. One exception to this was reported by Jane Goodall. This episode, the only one of its kind, occurred when a mature chimpanzee climbed a tree 10 feet above her head and worked himself into a rage, screaming and hitting the trunk. About 5 minutes later, he climbed down, moved behind her and, after a short yell, hit her on the head. She did not witness any other severe persistent attack behavior that resulted in serious injury or death of another member of the group. One wonders whether a brain investigation in this chimpanzee would have revealed damage in the limbic system.

Another large-brained mammal, the dolphin, has been investigated by John Lilly. He suggested that dolphins have a high degree of control over their behavior, as do the related whales. An investigation of cases in which the ferocious sperm whale was said to have attacked whaling vessels in the 19th century was of interest. In six cases that were available for detailed scrutiny, the author was able to check the original handwritten logs of the ships. He found that the attack of the sperm whale was provoked in every instance by prior human attack, for in in every one of these cases, the whales had been wounded by a harpoon.

Conclusion

To sum up then, many biologists (and especially ethologists) consider the human particularly susceptible to violent behavior as compared to other animal species. Simply stated the logic of their argument is:

1. The predatory animals, e.g., wolves and lions, had to evolve instinctual control mechanisms to prevent intraspecies annihilation because they were so heavily armed with teeth and claws.

2. Prey animals such as rabbits and doves, not so armed, but well equipped to flee, had no need to develop these control mechanisms. In confined quarters, however, male competitiveness in these species will frequently lead to physical violence and murder.
3. Man is biologically unarmed and therefore without evolved, instinctual control mechanisms over violence. He is also in confined quarters with numerous diverse threats to his sense of territoriality.
4. Therefore, when man displays aggression toward another man, there are no internal checks on the limits to which he will go—only weak, learned, social controls are present.*

There are two key points in all these formulations. One is that man has an aggressive instinct, the extreme of which is personal violence resulting in homicide. The other is that he has failed to evolve the necessary cerebral control mechanisms to prevent this instinct from dominating behavior.

The evidence that we offer in this present book *does not support either of these contentions*. Aggression as defined in this argument is not a simple instinct, but one of a number of different varieties of behavior which are controlled and modulated at different levels of brain function. Even though the basic fight-or-flight brain mechanism may be used in the complex behavioral patterns of aggressive violence, the patterns themselves are learned and the basic mechanisms are significantly altered. Furthermore, powerful cerebral mechanisms do exist which in extreme cases can stop directed attack behavior in midcharge. We therefore deny that a normal man in a one-to-one relationship with another human being is more prone to violence than the individual of any other species.

However, if man's brain is diseased or malfunctioning, then

* A modified version of this position has been offered by Anthony Storr in *Human Aggression*. He proposes that the biological constraints are present, as evidenced by the fact that most humans avoid kicking an enemy when he is down or will even offer help to a wounded enemy in war time. He suggests, however, that a social problem has been created by the increasing distance between modern armies made possible by modern technology. He argues that the pushing of a button producing millions of deaths does not have the same power that a bleeding human does to stop violence by exciting biological control mechanisms. We would agree with this important insight.

his capacity for senseless violence exceeds that of any other animal, for his repertoire of behavior and his lethal abilities surpass those of other species. Let us in the following chapters review the kinds of abnormalities that occur in the human brain, with their possible consequences as far as violent behavior is concerned.

REFERENCES

Adams, D., and Flynn, J. P. Transfer of an escape response from tail shock to brain stimulated attack behavior. *J. Exp. Anal. Behav. 9:*401–408, 1966.

Alonso deFlorida, F., and Delgado, J. M. R. Lasting effects on behavior evoked by cerebral stimulation of the cat. *Amer. J. Physiol. 183:*592, 1955.

Alonso de Florida, F., and Delgado, J. M. R. Lasting behavioral and EEG changes in cats induced by prolonged stimulation of amygdala. *Amer. J. Physiol. 193:*223–229, 1958.

Anand, B. K., and Brobeck, J. R. Food intake and spontaneous activity of rats with lesions in the amygdoid nuclei. *J.Neurophysiol.* 15:424–480, 1952.

Anand, B. K., and Dua, S. Stimulation of limbic system of brain in waking animals. *Science* 122:1139, 1955.

Anand, B. K., and Dua, S. Electrical stimulation of the limbic system of brain ("visceral brain") in the waking animals. *Indian J. Med. Res. 44:*107–119, 1956.

Anand, B. K., Dua, S., and Chhina, G. S. Changes in the affective behavior produced by lesions in the frontal and temporal lobes. *Indian J. Med. Res. 45:*353–357, 1957.

Anand, B. K., Chhina, G. S., and Dua, S. Effects of lesions in the limbic system on the affective behavior and visceral responses in monkeys and cats. *Indian J. Med. Res. 47:*51–58, 1959

Anderson, O. D. The role of the glands of internal Secretion in the production of behavioral types in the dog. Section VII In: *The Genetic and Endocrine Basis for Differences in Form and Behavior* (C. R. Stockard, ed.). *Mem., 19:*647–747, 1941.

Arana-Iniguez, R., Reis, D. J., Naquet, R., and Magoun, H. W. Propagation of amygdaloid seizures. *Acta Neural. Latinoam. 1:*109–122, 1955.

Ardrey, R. *The Territorial Imperative.* New York, Atheneum, 1966.

Bard, P. A diencephalic mechanism for the expression of rage, with special reference to the sympathetic nervous system. *Amer. J. Physiol. 84:*490–515, 1928.

Bard, P., and Mountcastle, V. B. Some forebrain mechanisms involved in expression of rage: With special reference to suppression of angry behavior. *Res. Nerv. Ment. Dis. Proc.* 27:362–404, 1948.

Bard, P. "Central Nervous Mechanisms for the Expression of Anger in Animals." In: *Feelings and Emotions: The Mooseheart Symposium* (M. L. Reymart, ed.). New York, McGraw-Hill, pp. 211–237, 1950.

Bargman, W., and Schadé, J. P., eds. *The Rhinencephalon and Related Structures: Progress in Brain Research, Vol. 3.* New York, Elsevier, 1963.

Beck, E., Meyer, A., and LeBeau, J. Efferent connexions of the human prefontal region with reference to fronto-hypothalamic pathways. *J. Neurol. Neurosurg. Psychiat. 14:*295–302, 1951.

Bente, D., and Kluge, E. Sexuelle Reizzustände im Rahmen des Uncinatus-Syndroms: Ein klinischer Beitrag zur Pathophysiologie und Pathobiologie des Archicortex. *Arch. Psychiat. 190:*357–376, 1953.

Brady, J. V., and Nauta, W. J. H. Subcortical mechanisms in emotional behavior: Affective changes following septal forebrain lesions in the albino rat. *J. Comp. Physiol. Psychol. 46:*339–346, 1953.

Brady, J. V., Schreiner, L., Geller, I., and Kling, A. Subcortical mechanisms in emotional behavior: The effect of rhinencephalic injury upon the acquisition and retention of a conditioned avoidance response in cats. *J. Comp. Physiol. Psychol. 47:*179–186, 1954.

Brady, J. V., and Nauta, W. J. H. Subcortical mechanisms in emotional behavior: The duration of affective changes following septal and habenular lesions in the albino rat. *J. comp. Physiol. Psychol., 48:*412–420, 1955.

Brady, J. V.: "Emotional Behavior." In: *Handbook of Physiology, Vol.* 3. (J. Field, H. W. Magoun, and V. E. Hall, Eds.) Washington, D.C., American Physiological Society, pp. 316–318, 1960.

Brunnell, B. N. The effects of septal and amygdaloid lesions on aggressiveness and social dominance in the hamster. Paper presented at the Annual Meeting of the Psychonomic Society, Chicago. October, 1965.

Brunnell, B. N., Bemporad, J. R. and Flesher, C. K. Septal forebrain lesions and social dominance behavior in the hooded rat. *Psychon. Sci. 6:*207–208, 1966.

Brunnell, B. N. Amygdaloid lesions and social dominance in the hooded rat. *Psychon. Sci. 6:*93–94, 1966.

Brunnell, B. N., and Smith, M. H. Septal lesions and aggressiveness in the cotton rat, sigmodon hispidus. *Psychon. Sci. 6:*443–444, 1966.

Buchwald, N. A., and Ervin, F. R. Evoked potentials and behavior: A study of responses to subcortical stimulation in the awake, unrestrained animal. *EEG Neurophysiol. 9:*477–496, 1957.

Bursten, B., and Delgado, J. M. R. Positive reinforcement induced by intracerebral stimulation in the monkey. *J. Comp. Physiol. Psychol.* *51*:6–10, 1958.

Cannon, W. B. *Bodily Changes in Pain, Hunger, Fear and Rage.* New York, Appleton-Century-Crofts, 1920.

Carpenter, C. R. "Territoriality: A Review of Concepts and Problems." In: *Behavior and Evolution* (A. Roe and Simpson, G. G., eds.). New Haven, Yale Univer. Press, 1958.

Carpenter, C. R. *Naturalistic Behavior of Non-Human Primates.* University Park, Pennsylvania State Univer. Press, 1964.

Carthy, J. D., and Ebling, F. J., eds. *The Natural History of Aggression.* New York, Academic Press, 1954.

Clark, L. D. "Experimental Studies of the Behavior of an Aggressive Predatory Mouse (Onychomys Leucogaster)." In: *Roots of Behavior* (E. L. Bliss ed.) New York, Hoeber, pp. 179–186, 1962.

Clemente, C. D., and Lindsey, D. B., eds. *Aggression and Defense. Neural Mechanisms and Social Patterns (Brain Function Vol. V.).* UCLA Forum in Medical Sciences, No. 7. Berkeley, Univ. of California Press, 1967.

Collias, N. E. Aggressive behavior among vertebrate animals. *Physiol. Zool. 17*:83–123, 1944.

Creutzfeldt, O. Spread of convulsions in the temporal lobe of the cat: Discharge of convulsions at cornu Ammonis and its relation to the other portions of the rhinencephalon and isocortex. *Schweiz. Arch. Neur. Psychiat. 77*:163–194, 1956.

DaVanzo, J. P., Daugherty, M., Ruckert, R. and Kang, L. Pharmacological and biochemical studies in isolation induced fighting in mice. *Psychopharmacologia 9*:210–219, 1966.

Davis, C. E.: "The Physiological Analysis of Aggressive Behavior." In *Social Behavior and Organization Among Vertebrates* (W. Etkin, ed.). Chicago, Univ. Chicago Press, pp. 53–74, 1964.

Delgado, J. M. R. Cerebral mechanisms possibly related to pain and fear. *Arch. Neurol. Psychiat. 73*:576, 1955.

Delgado, J. M. R., Rosvold, H. E., and Looney, E. Evoking conditioned fear by electrical stimulation of subcortical structures in the monkey brain. *J. Comp. Physiol. Psychol. 49*:373–380, 1956.

Delgado, J. M. R., and Bursten, B. Attraction and avoidance evoked by septal and rhinencephalic stimulation in the monkey. *Fed. Proc. 15*:45, 1956.

Delgado, J. M. R., Ushiyama, J., and Garotte, L. Effects of repeated cerebral stimulation in monkeys. *Fed. Proc. 17*:34, 1958.

Delgado, J. M. R., and Sevillano, M. Evolution of repeated hippocampal seizures in the cat. *EEG Clin. Neurophysiol. 13*:722–733, 1961.

DeMolina, A. F., and Hunsperger, R. W. Central representation of affective reactions in fore-brain and brain stem: Electrical stimulation of amygdala, stria terminalis, and adjacent structures. *J. Physiol. 145:*251–265, 1959.

DeVore, I. (ed.): *Primate Behavior.* New York, Holt, Rinehart and Winston, 1965.

Downer, J. L. deC. "Interhemispheric Integration in the Visual System." In: *Conference on Interhemispheric Relations and Cerebral Dominance* (V. B. Mountcastle, ed.). Baltimore, The Johns Hopkins Press, 1962, pp. 83–100.

Egger, M. D., and Flynn, J. P. Effects of electrical stimulation of the amygdala on hypothalamically elicited attack behavior in cats. *J. Neurophysiol. 26:*705–720, 1963.

Egger, M. D., and Flynn, J. P. Further Studies of Amygdaloid Stimulations and Ablation on Hypothalamically Elicited Attack Behavior in Cats." In: *Structure and Function of the Limbic System, Vol.* 27, *Progress in Brain Research* (W. R. Adey and T. Tokizane, eds.). New York, Elsevier, 1967, pp. 165–182.

Eibl-Eibesfeldt, I. The fighting behavior of animals. *Sci. Amer. 205:*112–122, 1961.

Flynn, J. P., Wasman, M. and Egger, D. "Behavior During Propagated Hippocampal After-discharges." In: *EEG and Behavior* (G. H. Glaser, ed.). New York, Basic Books, pp. 134–148, 1963.

Fonberg, E., and Delgado, J. M. R. Avoidance and alimentary reactions during amygdala stimulation. *J. Neurophysiol. 24:*651–664, 1961.

Fuller, J. L., Rosvold, H. E., and Pribram, K. H. The effect on affective and cognitive behavior in the dog of lesions of the pyriform-amygdala-hippocampal complex. *J. Comp. Physiol. Psychol. 50:*89–96, 1957.

Gastaut, H., Vigouroux, R., Corriol, J., and Badier, M. Effects de la stimulation electrique (par electrodes a demeure) du complexe amygdalien chez le chat non narcose. *J. Physiol. (Paris) 43:*740–746, 1951.

Gastaut, H., Naquet, R., Vigouroux, R. and Corriol, J. Provocation de comportements émotionnels divers par stimulation rhinencéphalique chez le chat avec électrodes à demeure. *Rev. Neurol. 86:*319–327, 1952.

Gastaut, H., Terzian, H., Naquet, R. and Luschnat, K. Correlations entres les "automatismes" des crises temporales et la phénomènes electroencéphalographiques qui les accompagnent. *Rev. Neurol. 86:*678–682, 1952.

Gastaut, H., Vigouroux, R., and Naquet, R. Comportements posturaux et cinétiques provoques par stimulation sous-corticale chez le chat non anesthésié. *J. Psychol. Norm. Path. 45:*257–271, 1952.

Gastaut, H. Correlations entre le système nerveux négétatif et le système de la vie de relation dans el rhinencéphale. *J. Physiol. (Paris) 44:*431–470, 1952.

Gastaut, H., Naquet, R., Vigouroux, R., Roger, A., and Badier, M. Etude électrographique chez l'homme et chez l'animal des décharges épileptiques dites "psychomotrices." *Rev. Neurol. 88:*310–354, 1953.

Gastaut, H., Naquet, R., and Roger, A. Etude des postdécharges électriques provoquées par stimulation du complexe nucléaire amygdalien chez la rat. *Rev. Neurol. 87:*224–231, 1952.

Gastaut, H., Naquet, R. and Vigouroux, R. Un cas d'épilepsie amygdalienne expérimentale chez le chat. *EEG Clin. Neurophysiol. 5:*291–294, 1953.

Gastaut, H., Vigouroux, R., and Naquet, R. Lésions épileptogènes amygadalo-hippocampiques provoquées chez le chat par injection de "crème d'alumine." *Rev. Neurol. 87:*607–609, 1952.

Gless, P., Cole, J., Whitty, C., and Cairns, H. The effects of lesions in the cingular gyrus and adjacent areas in monkeys. *J. Neurol. Neurosurg. Psychiat. 13:*178–190, 1950.

Gloor, P. Electrophysiological studies on connections of amygdaloid nucleus in cat: Electrophysiological properties of amygdaloid projection system. *EEG Clin. Neurophysiol. 7:*243–264, 1955.

Gloor, P. The pattern of conduction of amygdaloid seizure discharge: An experimental study in the cat. *Arch. Neur. Psychiat. 77:*247–258, 1957.

Gloor, P. "Amygdala." In: *Handbook of Physiology,* Sec. 1., Neurophysiology, Vol. II (John Field, ed. in chief). Washington, D.C., American Physiology Society, 1960, pp. 1395–1520.

Goddard, G. V. Function of the amygdala. *Psychol. Bull. 62:*89–109, 1964.

Goodall, J. Chimpanzees of Combe Stream Reserve. In: *Primate Behavior* (I. DeVore, ed.) New York, Holt, Rinehart and Winston, 1965, p. 425.

Green, J. D., Clemente, C. D., and deGroot, J. Rhinencephalic lesions and behavior in cats. *J. Comp. Neurol. 108:*505–536, 1957.

Heath, R. G., Monroe, R. R., and Mickle, W. Stimulation of the amygdaloid nucleus in a schizophrenic patient. *Amer. J. Psychiat. 111:*862–863, 1955.

Hunsperger, R. W. Affektreaktionen auf elektrische Reizung im Hirnstamm der Katze. *Helvet Physiol. Pharmacol. Acta. 14:*70, 1956.

Jasper, H., and Rasmussen, T. Studies of clinical and electrical responses to deep temporal stimulation in men with some considerations of functional anatomy. *Res. Nerv. Ment. Dis., Proc. 36:*316–334, 1958.

Kaada, B. R. Somato motor, autonomic and electrocortigraphic responses to electrical stimulation of "rhinencephalic" and other structures in primates, cat and dog: Study of responses from limbic, subcallosal, orbitoinsular, piriform and temporal cortex, hippocampus-fornix and amygdala. *Acta Physiol. scand. 24* (Suppl. 83): 1–285, 1951.

Kaada, B. R., Jansen, J., and Andersen, P. Stimulation of the hippocompus and medial cortical areas in unanesthetized cats. *Neurology 3:*843–857, 1953.

Kaada, B. R.: Temporal lobe seizures. *ECG Clin. Neurophysiol. (Suppl.) 4:*235–246, 1954.

Kaada, B. R., Andersen, P., and Jansen, J., Jr. Stimulation of the amygdaloid nuclear complex in unanesthetised cats. *Neurology, 4:*48–64, 1954.

Kaada, B. R.: "Cingulate, Posterior Orbital, Anterior Insular and Temporal Pole Cortex." In: *Handbook of Physiology, Sec. 1, Neurophysiology, Vol. II* (John Field, ed. in chief). Washington, D.C., American Physiology Society, 1960, pp. 1345–1372.

Kaada, B. Brain mechanisms related to aggressive behavior. In: *Aggression and Defense.* Los Angeles, UCLA Press, 1967.

Karli, P. Hormones steroides et comportement d'agression interspecifique rat-souris. *J. Physiol. Path. Gen. 50:*346–347, 1958.

Karli, P., and Vergnes, M. Nouvelles donnees sur les bases neurophysiologiques du comportement d'agression inter-specifique rat-souris. *J. Physiol. 56:*384, 1964.

Karli, P., and Vergnes, M. Role du rhinencephale dans le controle du comportement d'agression inter-specifique rat-souris. *J. Physiol. 55:*272–273, 1963.

King, F. A. Effects of septal and amygdaloid lesions on emotional behavior and conditioned avoidance responses in the rat, *J. Nerv. Ment. Dis. 126:*57–63, 1958.

King, F. A., and Meyer, P. M. Effects of amygdaloid lesions upon septal hyper-emotionality in the rat. *Science 128:*655–656, 1958.

Kling, A., and Hutt, P. J. Effect of hypothalamic lesions on the amygdala syndrome in the cat, *Arch. Neurol. Psychiat. 79:*511–517, 1958.

Klüver, H., and Bucy, P. C. Psychic blindness and other symptoms following bilateral temporal lobectomy in rhesus monkeys. *Amer. J. Physiol. 119:*352–353, 1937.

Klüver, H., and Bucy, P. C. Preliminary analysis of functions of temporal lobes in monkeys. *Arch. Neurol. Psychiat., 42:*979–1000, 1939.

Kreiger, H. P., Kolodny, H., and Kreiger, D. T. Elicitation of sham rage by implantation of carbachol into the hypothalamus. *Fed. Proc. 22:*515. 1963.

Kuo, Z. Y. Studies on the basic factors in animal fighting: Part I–IV. *J. Genet. Psychol. 96:*201–239, 1960.

Levison, P. K., and Flynn, J. P. The objects attacked by cats during stimulation of the hypothalamus. *Animal Behaviour 13:*217–220, 1965.

Lilly, J. C. *The Mind of the Dolphin.* New York, Doubleday, 1967.

Lorenz, K. *On Aggression.* New York, Harcourt, Brace & World, 1966.

MacDonnell, M. F., and Flynn, J. P. Attack elicited by stimulation of the thalamus of cats. *Science 144:*1249–1250, 1964.

MacLean, P. D. Some psychiatric implications of physiological studies on frontotemporal portion of limbic system (visceral brain). *EEG Clin. Neurophysiol. 4:*407–418, 1952.

MacLean, P. D., and Delgado, J. M. R. Electrical and chemical stimulation of frontotemporal portion of limbic system in the waking animal. *EEG Clin. Neurophysiol. 5:*91–100, 1953.

Marler, P., and Hamilton, W. J., III *Mechanisms of Animal Behavior.* New York, Wiley, 1966.

Meyer, A., and Beck, E. The hippocampal formation in temporal lobe epilepsy. *Proc. Roy. Soc. Med. 48:*457–462, 1955.

Montague, M. F. Ashley. *Man and Aggression.* New York, Oxford Univ. Press, 1968.

Morrell, F., Roberts, H. L., and Jasper, H. H. Effect of focal epileptogenic lesions and their ablation upon conditioned electrical responses of brain in monkey. *EEG Clin. Neurophysiol. 8:*217–236, 1956.

Morin, G., Gastaut, H., Vigouroux, R., and Roger, A. Comportement émotionnel et lésions expérimentales du rhinencéphale chez le chat. *C. R. Soc. Biol. 146:*1959–1961, 1952.

Morin, G., Gastaut, H., Vigouroux, R., and Naquet, R. Reproduction expérimentale de l'épilepsie de type "psycho-moteur" chez le chat. *C. R. Acad. Sci. (Paris) 235:*1561–1562, 1952.

Morris, D. *The Naked Ape.* London, Jonathan Cape, 1967.

Moyer, K. E. *Kinds of Aggression and Their Physiological Basis. Report No. 67–12.* Pittsburgh, Carnegie-Mellon Univer.

Myer, J. S., and White R. T. Aggressive motivation in the rat. *Animal Behaviour, 13:*430–433, 1965.

Nakao, H. Emotional behavior produced by hypothalamic stimulation. *Amer. J. Physiol. 194:*411–418, 1958.

Naquet, R. *Sur les fonctions du rhinencephale d'apres les resultats de sa stimulation chez le chat* (Thesis). Marseille, 1953.

Papez, J. W. A proposed mechanism of emotion. *Arch. Neurol. Psychiat. 38:*725–743, 1937.

Pavlov, I. P. *Lectures on Conditioned Reflexes* (W. H. Gantt, trans.) New York: International, p. 414, 1928.

Poirier, L. J. Anatomical and experimental studies on the temporal pole of the Macaques. *J. Comp. Neurol. 96:*209–248, 1952.

Pribram, K. H., and Bagshaw, M. Further analysis of the temporal lobe syndrome utilizing fronto-temporal ablations. *J. Comp. Neurol. 99:*347–375, 1953.

Ramey, E. R., and O'Doherty, D. S. (eds.). *Electrical Studies on the Unanesthetized Brain.* New York, Hoeber, 1960.

Roberts, W. W., and Kiess, H. O. Motivational properties of hypothalamic aggression in cats. *J. Comp. Physiol. Psychol. 58:*187–193, 1964.

Robinson, B. W., and Mishkin, M. Penile erection evoked from forebrain structures in Macaca mulatta. *Arch. Neurol. 19:*184-198, 1968.

Rodriguez Delgado, R., and Delgado, J. M. R. An objective approach to measurement of behavior. *Phil. Sci. 29:*253–268, 1962.

Rosner, B. S., Goff, W. R., and Allison, T. "Cerebral Electrical Responses to External Stimuli." In *EEG and Behavior* (G. H. Glaser, ed.). New York, Basic Books, pp. 109–133, 1963.

Rosvold, H. E., Mirsky, A. F., and Pribram, K. H. Influence of amygdalectomy on social behavior in monkeys. *J. Comp. Physiol. Psychol. 47:*173–178, 1954.

Rosvold, H. E., and Delgado, J. M. R. Effect of electrical stimulation of the brain on the behavior of monkeys. *Proc. 14th Int. Congr. Psychol.* pp. 163–164, 1954.

Schreiner, L. H., and Kling, A. A behavioral change following rhinencephalic injury in the cat. *J. Neurophysiol. 16:*643–659, 1953.

Schreiner, L. H., and Kling, A. Effects of castration on hypersexual behavior induced by rhinencephalic injury in cat. *Arch. Neurol. Psychiat. 72:*180–186, 1954.

Simma, K. Die psychischen Storüngen bei Läsionen des Temporallappens und ihre Behandlung: Eine elektroencephalographischklinische und pathologisch-anatomische Studie. *Monatsschr. Psychiat. Neurol.* 130:129–160, 1955.

Smith, W. K. Non-olfactory function of the pyriform-amygdaloid-hippocampal complex. *Fed. Proc. 9:*118, 1950.

Spiegel, E. A., Miller, H. R., and Oppenheimer, M. J. Forebrain and rage reactions. *J. Neurophysiol. 3:*538–548, 1940.

Thomson, A. F., and Walker, A. E. Behavioral alterations following lesions of the medial surface of the temporal lobe. *Folia Psychiat. Neerl. 53:*444–452, 1950.

Tinbergen, N. Fighting and threat in animals. *New Biology 14:*9–24, 1953.

Tolman, J., and King, J. A. The effects of testosterone propionate on aggression in male and female C57BL/10 mice. *Brit. J. Anim. Behav. 4:*147–149, 1956.

Ursin, H., and Kaada, B. Functional localization within the amygdaloid complex in the cat. *EEG Clin. Neurophysiol. 12:*1–20, 1960.

Vigouroux, R., Gastaut, H., and Badier, M. Les formes expérimentales de l'épilepsie. *Rev. neurol. 85:*505–508, 1951.

Walker, A. E., Thompson, A. F., and McQueen, J. D. Behavior and the temporal rhinencepholon in the monkey. *Bull. Johns Hopkins Hosp. 93:*65–93, 1953.

Wasman, M., and Flynn, J. P. Directed attack elicited from hypothalmus. *Arch. Neurol. 6:*220–227, 1962.

Weiskrantz, L. Behavioral changes associated with ablation of the amygdaloid complex in monkeys. *J. Comp. Physiol. Psychol. 49:*381–394, 1956.

Wheatley, M. D. The hypothalamus and affective behavior in cats. *Arch. Neurol. Psychiat. 52:*296–316, 1944.

Wood, C. D. Behavioral changes following discrete lesions of temporal lobe structures. *Neurology* (Supp. 1) *8:*215–220, 1958.

Woods, J. W. "Taming" of the wild Norway rat by rhinencephalic lesions. *Nature (London) 178:*869, 1956.

Yasukochi, G. Emotional responses elicited by electrical stimulation of the hypothalamus in cat. *Folia Psychiat. Neurol. Japonica 14:*260–267, 1960.

Yen, H. C. Y., Day, C. A., and Sigg, E. B. Influence of endocrine factors on development of fighting behavior in rodents. *Pharmacologist 4:*173, 1962.

Zuckerman, S. *The Social Life of Monkeys and Apes.* London, Kegan Paul, 1932.

Chapter 4

Genetic Brain Disease

We are truly heirs of all the ages; but as honest men it behooves us to learn the extent of our inheritance, and as brave ones not to whimper if it should prove less than we had supposed.

John Tyndall

Fragments of Science, Volume II,
Matter and Force

The evidence from animal experiments, as well as data from human patients (to be described in Chapter 7), support the idea that individual violence may be one of the symptoms of a disturbance in the brain mechanisms that control, initiate, and suppress violent behavior. These mechanisms can be disturbed by brain disease—both acquired (as from a blow on the head) and genetic.

In spite of statistical evidence which showed that abnormal behavior occurred much more often in both identical twins than in both fraternal twins, if one of the twins was known to exhibit this kind of behavior, the association of behavioral changes with inheritance has not been accepted by most behavioral scientists. They, in fact, felt that the older simplistic theories of inherited antisocial behavior were thoroughly discredited. However, the new techniques of cytogenetics, which permit us to see the chromosomes that carry genetic information within every cell have made it possible to describe an individual in terms of his genetic structure; these techniques have also allowed us to begin to correlate abnormalities in the genes with observed abnormal behavior, including mental deficiency, antisocial behavior, and violence.

The genes are submicroscopic particles that dictate skin and eye color, body build, and other inherited characteristics; they are located in oblong structures—the chromosomes—within the nucleus of every cell in the body. In each normal human cell, there are 46 chromosomes, or 23 pairs, and the conventional way to refer to them is with the letters of the alphabet. Each pair is made up of one chromosome from the fertilizing sperm of the father and one from the egg of the mother. Two of these chromosomes, the so-called X and Y chromosomes, determine sex. A woman normally has two Xs as her pair of sex chromosomes, and a man's pair is made up of one X and one Y. The other 22 chromosome pairs are called autosomes.

Chromosomal or cytogenetic abnormalities are not by any means necessarily inherited. They may occur in the fetus any time a cell divides—which is to say, they may represent an injury to the chromosomes after conception. The earlier any such injury occurs the more widespread will the resulting disorder be in a developing infant.

One kind of genetic abnormality known to produce maldevelopment is the appearance of extra chromosomes within one of the 23 pairs, so that instead of the normal two, an individual has three or four. As every cell in the body has the same number of chromosomes, (unless a "focal aneuploidy" occurs late after conception—e.g., a harelip or cleft palate) these abnormalities can be discovered by examining cells cells for this purpose are usually taken from the blood stream or from the mucous membrane of the mouth. Triplication or "trisomy" within the G, D, or E pairs of autosomes, for instance, seriously disturbs brain development. Triplication of the G autosomes causes mongolism; triplication of the D autosomes means that the two brain hemispheres will fail to separate and that the "nose brain" does not develop at all; a triplication of the E autosomes means that the entire brain fails to develop and the head is extremely small. A child with brain defects produced by these last two genetic abnormalities usually will not live more than a few months.

Alterations in the sex chromosomes are associated with less severe disruptions of brain function and behavior than autosomal trisomy. An extra Y (male) chromosome in a woman seems to be related to a masculine type of body build and musculature; an attempt was made not long ago to discredit the performance of outstanding women athletes on the grounds that as "XXYs," they were not completely female. But in fact the presence of one or two extra X chromosomes may have more serious implications for a woman than the presence of an extra Y; statistical studies have shown that XXX women are more likely to be mentally deficient than women with the normal complement of two X chromosomes.

The addition of one or two extra X chromosomes in the male, producing an XXY or XXXY configuration, is often associated with impaired genital development, as well as with speech and reading difficulties. In 1953, Zublin noted that men with the XXY chromosomal configuration tend to exhibit antisocial behavior. Since then a number of investigators have tested large groups for genetic abnormalities, and found that although no more than 0.2% of male infants in the general population have an extra X chromosome, the XXY abnormality occurs more than 20 times as often in the male inmates of criminal and mental institutions. The XYY configuration also seems to be related to antisocial behavior, especially violence. One study of male prison inmates who showed violent behavior revealed an unusual incidence of the XYY chromosomal pattern. Many XYY men tend to be taller than their siblings and are more apt to start displaying intractable antisocial behavior at a very early age. This study also compared a group of XYY offenders with another group of violent prisoners of similar ages, intelligences, and social backgrounds, but with a normal XY chromosome pattern. The violent XY males usually had siblings who had broken the law, whereas the XYY males were more likely to have come from law-abiding families. XYY males were reported to be more apt to destroy property than human beings, although assaults on other people were far from rare. These subjects were more refractory to social rehabilitation than the XYs.

Only a small percentage of violent offenders are XYY males, and we are not implying that all XYY men are violent or antisocial. The point we are making by referring to these studies is that as the chromosomes themselves do not directly influence actions, the disturbed behavior of XYY males must be related to altered brain function. The XYY configuration may be only a signal of possible brain malfunction.

We need to study XYY males to find out much more than we now know about the behavioral implications of chromosomal abnormalities. Since the duplicated chromosome is a sex chromosome, does it in fact result in an abnormal hormonal level in the blood that bathes the brain cells? If there is in fact such an altered level, can it be associated with unusual or abnormal behavior? Are these abnormal sex chromosomes related to any other easily detectable change in body pattern? There is some recent evidence, for instance, that the fingerprint pattern may be affected by chromosomal reduplication, and that certain forms of fingerprint abnormalities are particularly prevalent among individuals convicted of committing sexual crimes.

We also need to know a great deal more about brain function itself in XYY individuals. As we have suggested, there may be some structural abnormalitiy of the brain—particularly of the limbic system—which is characteristic of the XYY inheritance. Thus, thorough investigations of brain function in all XYY males, whether violent or not, should be carried out. Such studies may have far reaching significance because they could form a model for more extensive investigations and correlations of other genetic abnormalities with abnormal behavior.

REFERENCES

Anderson, I. F., Goeller, E. A., and Wallace, C. Sex chromosome abnormalities in a population of 1,662 mental defectives. *S. Afr. Med. J. 38:*346–349, 1964.

Barr, M. L., and Hobbs, B. E. Chromosomal sex in transvestites. *Lancet 1:*1109–1110, 1954.

Benda, C. E. *Mongolism and Cretinism.* New York, Grune & Stratton, 1949.

Boczowski, K., and Casey, M. D. Pattern of DNA replication of the sex chromosomes in three males, two with XYY and one with XXYY karyotype. *Nature 213:*928–930, 1967.

Carr, D. H., Barr, M. L., and Plunkett, E. R. An XXXX sex chromosome complex in two mentally defective females. *Canad. Med. Ass. J. 84:* 131–137, 1961.

Casey, M. D., Blank, C. E., Street, D. R. K., Segall, L. J., McDougall, J. H., McGrath, P. J., and Skinner, J. L. YY chromosomes and antisocial behavior. *Lancet 2:*859–860, 1966.

Casey, M. D., Segall, L. J., Street, D. R., and Blank, C. E. Sex chromosome abnormalities in two state hospitals for patients requiring special security. *Nature 209:*641–642, 1966.

Court-Brown, W. M., Jacobs, P. A., and Brunton, M. Chromosome studies of randomly chosen men and women. *Lancet* 2:561, 1965.

Danon, M., and Sachs, L. Sex chromosomes and human sexual development. *Lancet 11:*20–25, 1957.

Darke, R. A. Heredity as etiological factor in homosexuality. *J. Nerv. Ment. Dis. 107:*251–268, 1948.

De La Chapelle, A. Sex chromosome abnormalities among mentally defectives in Finland. *J. Ment. Defic. Res.* 7:129–139, 1963.

Ferguson-Smith, M. A. Chromatin-positive Klinefelter's syndrome (primary micro-orchidism) in a mental-deficiency hospital. *Lancet 1:*928–931, 1958.

Ferguson-Smith, M. A. The prepubertal testicular lesion in chromatin-positive Klinefelter's syndrome (primary micro-orchidism) as seen in mentally handicapped children. *Lancet 1:*219–222, 1959.

Ferguson-Smith, M. A. Sex chromatin anomalies in mentally defective individuals. *Acta Cytol. (Phila.)* 6:73–83, 1962.

Forssman, H., and Hambert, G. Incidence of Klinefelter's syndrome among mental patients. *Lancet 1:*1327, 1963.

Fraser, J. H., Campbell, J. MacGilloray, R. C., Boyd, E., and Lennox, B. The XXX syndrome frequency among mental defectives and fertility. *Lancet* 2:626–627, 1960.

Gentele, H., Lagerholm, B., and Lodin, A. The chromosomal sex of male homosexuals. *Acta Dermat. 40:*470–473, 1960.

Goodman, R. M., Smith W. S., and Migeon, C. J. Sex chromosome abnormalities. *Nature 216:*942–943, 1967.

Hambert, G., and Frey, T. S. The electroencephalogram in the Klinefelter syndrome. *Acta Psychiat. Scand. 40:*28–36, 1964.

Hambert, G. *Males with Positive Sex Chromatin.* Copenhagen, Munksgaard, 1966.

Hamerton, J. L., Jagiello, G. M., and Kirman, B. H. Sex-chromosome abnormalities in a population of mentally defective children. *Brit. Med. J.* 5273:220–223, 1962.

Harnden, D. G., Jacobs, P. A., MacLean, N., and Mantle, D. J. Abnormalities of the sex chromosome complement in man. *Med. Res. J.:* (Report #305) 1964.

Hope, K., Philip, A. E., and Loughran, J. M. Psychological characteristics associated with XYY sex-chromosome complement in a state mental hospital. *Brit. J. Psychiat. 113:*495–498, 1967.

Hunter, H. Chromatin-positive and XYY boys in approved schools. *Lancet 1:*816, 1968.

Ismail, A. A., Harkness, R. A., Kirkham, K. E., Lordine, J. A., Whatmore, P. B., and Britton, R. P. Effect of abnormal sex-chromosome complements on urinary testosterone levels. *Lancet 1:*220–222, 1968.

Israelsohn, W. J., and Taylor, A. I. Chromatin-positive presumed Klinefelter's syndrome: Survey of boys in London schools for educationally subnormal children. *Brit. Med. J. 5226:*633–635, 1961.

Jacobs, P. A., Court-Brown, W. M., and Doll, R. Distribution of human chromosome counts in relation to age. *Nature 191:*1178–1180, 1961.

Jacobs, P. A., Brunton, M., and Court-Brown, W. M. Cytogenetic studies of leucocytes on the general population: Subject of ages 65 years or more. *Ann. Hum. Genet., 27:*353, 1964.

Jacobs, P. A., Brunton, M., Melville, M. M., Brittain, R. P., and McClemont, W. F. Aggressive behavior, mental sub-normality and the XYY male. *Nature 208:*1351, 1965.

Jacobs, P. A., Price, W. H., Court-Brown, W. M., Brittain, R. P., and Whatmore, P. B. Chromosome studies on men in a maximum security hospital. *Ann. Human Genet.* 1970, in press.

Kallman, F. J. Twin and sibship study of overt male homosexuality. *Amer. J. Human Genet. 4:*136–146, 1952.

Lang, T. Studies on genetic determinations of homosexuality. *J. Nerv. Ment. Dis. 92:*55–64, 1940.

Lang, T. Homosexuality as a genetic problem. *Acta. Genet. Med. (Roma) 9:*370–381, 1960.

Levij, I. S., Schaik, G. T., *et al.* Determination of genetic sex in homosexuals. *Nederl. Tijdsch. Geneesk. 100:*2121–2124, 1956.

Levine, S. Sex differences in the brain. *Sci. Amer. 214:*84–90, 1966.

Levine, S., and Conner, R. L. Endocrine Aspects of Violence. Report submitted to the National Commission on the Causes and Prevention of Violence, 1968.

Lubs, H. A. Testicular size in Klinefelter's syndrome in men over fifty: Report of a case with XXY/XY mosaicism. *New Eng. J. Med. 267:*326–331, 1962.

MacLean, N., Hardon, D. G., and Court-Brown, W. M. Abnormalities of sex chromosome constitution in newborn babies. *Lancet 2:*406–408, 1961.

MacLean, N., and Mitchell; J. M. A survey of sex-chromosome abnormalities among 4514 mental defectives. *Lancet 1:*293–296, 1962.

Marin-Padilla, M., Hoefnagel, D., and Benirschke, K. Anatomic and histopathologic study of two cases of D1(13–15) trisomy. *Cytogenet. 3:*258–284, 1964.

Marinello, M. J., Berkson, R. A., Edwards, J. A., and Bannerman, R. M. A study of the XYY syndrome in tall men and juvenile delinquents. JAMA *208:*321–325, 1969.

Mellbin, G. Neuropsychiatric disorders in six chromatin negative women. *Brit. J. Psychiat. 112:*145–148, 1966.

Michael, R. P. *Pathology and Treatment of Sexual Deviation.* London, Oxford Univ. Press, 1964.

Miller, O. J. The sex chromosome anomalies. *Amer. J. Obstet. Gynec. 90* (Suppl.): 1078–1139, 1964.

Money, J., Hampson, J., and Hampson, J. L. Examination of some basic sexual concepts: evidence of human hermaphroditism. *Bull. Johns Hopkins Hosp. 97:*301–319, 1955.

Money, J. Two cytogenetic syndromes: Psychologic comparisons: 1. Intelligence and specific-factor quotients. *J. Psychiat. Res. 2:*223–231, 1963.

Money, J. Cytogenic and psychosexual incongruities with a note on space-form blindness. *Amer. J. Psychiat. 119:*820–827, 1963.

Money, J., and Alexander, D. Turner's syndrome: Further demonstration of the presence of specific cognitional deficiencies. *J. Med. Genet. 3:*47–48, 1966.

Moor, L. Niveau intellectuel et polygonsomie: Confrontation du caryotype et du niveau mental de 374 malades dont le caryotype comporte un excès de chromosomes X ou Y. *Rev. Neuropsychiat. Infant 15:*325–348, 1967.

Mosier, H. D., Scott, L. W., and Cotter, L. H. The frequency of the positive sex-chromatin pattern in males with mental deficiency. *Pediatrics 25:*291–297, 1960.

Nielson, J. Prevalence of Klinefelter's syndrome in patients with mental disorders. *Lancet 1:*1109, 1964.

Pare, C. M. B. Homosexuality and chromosomal sex. *J. Psychosom. Res. 1:*247–251, 1956.

Price, W. H., Strong, J. A., Whatmore, P. B. and McClemont, W. F. Criminal patients with XYY sex chromosome complement. *Lancet 1:*565–566, 1966.

Pritchard, M. Homosexuality and genetic sex. *J. Ment. Sci. 108:*616–623, 1962.

Rabock, J., and Nedoma, K. Sex chromatin and sexual behavior: A study of 36 men with female nuclear pattern and of 194 homosexuals. *Psychosom. Med. 20:*55–59, 1958.

Razavi, L., Newell, J., and Droge, A. An approach to automatic counting of human metaphase chromosomes. (In press).

Razavi, L., Kozol, H., and Garafalo, R. Sex and other chromosomal anomalies among sexual criminals. (In press).

Shaffer, J. W. A specific cognitive deficit observed in gonadal aplasia (Turner's syndrome). *J. Clin. Psychol. 18:*402–406, 1962.

Shapiro, A., and Ridler, M. A. C. The incidence of Klinefelter's syndrome in a mental deficiency hospital. *J. Ment. Defic. Res. 4*:48–50, 1960.

Slater, E. In: *Symposium on Nuclear Sex* (D. R. Smith and W. M. Davidson, eds.). London, Heinemann, 1959, p. 79.

Taylor, A. I. Patau's, Edwards' and cri du chat syndromes: A tabulated summary of current findings. *Develop. Med. Child Neurol. 9*:78–86, 1967.

Telfer, M. A. Incidence of gross chromosomal errors among tall criminal American males. *Science 159*:1249–1250, 1968.

Torre, M. P. Discussion: Sociocultural factors in mental illness. *Ann. NY Acad. Sci. 84*:1921–1030, 1960.

Townes, P. L., Ziegler, N. A., and Leonard, L. W. A patient with 48 chromosomes (XXYY). *Lancet 1*:1041–1043, 1965.

Wegman, T. G., and Smith, D. W. Incidence of Klinefelter's syndrome among juvenile delinquents and felons. *Lancet 1*:274, 1963.

Wiener, S., Sutherland, G., Bartholomew, A. A., and Hudson, B. XYY males in a Melbourne prison. *Lancet 1*:150, 1968.

Yakovlev, P. I. Motility, behavior and brain; stereodynamic organizations and neural coordinates of behavior. *J. Nerv. Ment. Dis. 107*:313–335, 1948.

Zublin, O. Zur psychologie des Klinefelter Syndrome. *Acta Endocrinologica 14*:137–144, 1953.

Chapter 5

Acquired Brain Disease and Violence

Of Dog Madness (in Man)

Afterwards doth everything consistently grow worse and you'll soon see him loll out his rough tongue, gape wide, speak hoarse and have a great drought; grow raving at every attempt to drink, at the sight or touch of any liquor, gather froth in and about his mouth; to endeavor the spitting of the same upon the bystanders, even against his will; he gnashes his teeth with froth—snarling like a dog; his pulse now and breathing begins to fail, cold sweats break out on all sides, raves in the highest degree, not withstanding which he is all the while sensible and is afraid for the bystanders that he shall unwillingly hurt them.

The Aphorisms of Boerhaave
translated by Delacoste, 1715

The genetic abnormalities discussed in Chapter 4 occur in the fertilized egg and the growing fetus—in other words, before the brain has assumed its final form. Of course the brain also can be damaged and its functioning disrupted after it is fully formed. The later any such affliction strikes, the easier it is to observe the ensuing changes of previous behavior patterns (e.g., the behavioral change produced by a brain tumor in a 40-year-old man is easier to spot than the change in a 2-year-old child with the same disorder). The relationship between nongenetic brain disease (especially of the limbic brain) to the overt symptoms of abnormal or violent behavior is thus a relatively obvious matter, and one that is well-documented by centuries of medical observation. Uncontrolled violent behavior is known to be one of the symptoms of structural brain damage that can be due to lack of oxygen, head injury, viral infection, and tumors. In addition, violent and aggressive behavior may occur as the result of a functional abnormality of the brain—that is, it may be one of the symptoms associated with certain kinds of epilepsy even when brain structure is apparently normal.

Structural Brain Damage

A ready supply of oxygen is at all times an absolute prerequisite for normal brain function. Should this supply ever fail, the limbic system and especially the cells of the hippocampus are endangered. The hazards of oxygen insufficiency are especially great at the time of birth. Although anesthesia has unquestionably done much to relieve maternal suffering during childbirth, excessive anesthesia may deprive the infant of needed oxygen during the crucial moments of delivery. If a prolonged lack of oxygen causes the death of brain cells, the child can suffer some degree of mental deficiency, cerebral palsy, or epilepsy.* Subtle damage may become apparent only later: sitting, standing, walking, and talking may be delayed long past the appropriate chronological ages; there may be continuing inability to control bowels and bladder; or, the child may be hyperkinetic—that is, exhibit impulsive hyperactivity quite resistant to social control.

* Lack of oxygen is merely one cause of brain damage in newborns. Maternal infections affecting the fetus, prolonged reduction in blood sugar, severe disproportion between the size of the mother's pelvis and the size of the baby's head, Rh incompatibility, and physical damage to the baby's head during delivery are other conditions that may produce mentally defective, epileptic, and paralytic (as well as hyperkinetic and violent) children.

Good prenatal care, competent obstetrics, and good postnatal nutrition would reduce the load of cerebral palsy, epilepsy, and mental retardation by an estimated 10 to 15 per cent, or more.

The typical severe hyperkinetic brain-injured child is indiscriminately aggressive and impulsively violent. He may keep in constant and socially disruptive motion—running, shouting, and destroying any object that he gets his hands on. Although some of these children have near normal intelligence, they are not educable. Their hyperactive antisocial behavior is too destructive for any organized schoolroom activity, and their attention span is usually so limited that they are unable to participate in any learning experience. For some of these children—even those whose brain damage is so widespread that there are areas of cell destruction in the cortex as well as in part of the limbic system—amphetamine drugs have occasionally helped reduce their frantic restlessness and violence. For other children, however, drug therapy does not work; and surgeons such as Narabayashi in Japan have treated these patients by operating directly in the limbic system, destroying part or all of the nucleus amygdala. In a majority of the children so treated by Narabayashi, the hyperkinetic and assaultive behavior was reduced, and those of his patients who were capable of attending school showed an unexpected intellectual capacity.

Head injuries in growing children, adolescents, and adults are very likely to damage the undersurface of the frontal lobe and the tips of the temporal lobe—in other words, those parts of the limbic brain that lie closest to the bones of the skull. Normally, brain and bones are separated from each other by a cushion of fluid and a tough membrane. But if the head is struck hard enough, or if the body suddenly hits the ground with some force, the frontal and temporal lobes may be jarred against the base of the skull. The resulting damage to the brain stem is indicated by the loss of consciousness. It often happens, however, that when the brain stem recovers and consciousness returns, the injured person undergoes a period of uninhibited, aggressive, and combative behavior. Most severe head injuries produce fairly widespread damage, so that it is difficult to ascribe altered behavior to the dysfunction of a certain brain area, but studies of patients with injuries known to involve chiefly the temporal lobe indicate that these patients tend to be inappropriately combative—that is, they show the effects of limbic dysfunction.

Viral infections of the brain often are marked by behavioral change. The victims of the epidemic of encephalitis lethargica that occurred throughout the world after World War I showed many different behavioral symptoms, including reversal of sleep-

and-wake cycles, deterioration of intellectual capacity, episodic difficulty in controlling impulses, and antisocial and violent actions.

The classical example of a viral infection of the brain that produces changes in behavior is the virus encephalitis that causes rabies—a disease whose very name, *rage* in French, *rabia* in Italian, and *Wut* in German—means madness or rage. The early symptoms of rabies may include mental aberrations, sexual overindulgence and assault, alcoholism, and periods of violent rage; the disorder's final stages are marked by melancholy, extreme irritability, difficulty in swallowing and breathing, and convulsions. In animals afflicted with this disease, a prominent symptom is the occurrence of an extremely vicious, and uncontrolled attack of rage, which is why the cry of "mad dog" has always evoked such fear. The virus responsible for rabies often infects the medial portion of the temporal lobe with prominent virus inclusion bodies in the cells of the hippocampal area; that is to say, even though the rabies virus is found in many brain cells, it characteristically infects the limbic system of the brain.

A tumor of the limbic brain may also be responsible for an uncontrollable eruption of violence, hostility, and assault. One such case was that of Donald L., a short, muscular, 43-year-old man, who, when we first saw him in the hospital, was restrained by heavy fish netting. Even so, his behavior was impressively threatening. He snarled, showed his teeth, and lashed out with either arm or leg as soon as any attendant approached him. His wife and daughter were too frightened to give a detailed history. All they could say was that for no apparent reason he had taken a butcher knife and tried his best to kill them. They had called the police, who had observed Donald's garbled and inappropriate speech and promptly brought him to the hospital. Further questioning of his family elicited the information that Donald had undergone a genuine change in his personality over the previous 6 months, and that during this time, he had also complained of severe headaches and blurred vision. After a large dose of intramuscular sedation, he became quiet enough for a neurological examination to be made. The ophthalmoscope revealed that his optic nerve head was swollen and hemorrhagic, a condition that is usually caused by increased pressure within the head—often as a result of a crowding mass such as a tumor inside the brain case. Special x-ray films of the brain were then taken, and they confirmed that he had a tumor. It was underneath the right frontal lobe, pressing on the front portion of his temporal lobe as well; that is, the tumor pressed directly on the limbic system.

When the tumor was removed, Donald's symptoms disappeared and he peaceably went back to work as a night watchman.

Donald L.'s symptoms were not unusual for a man with a limbic brain tumor. Malamud's recent study of 18 people with tumors of the limbic brain revealed that all had some psychiatric disorder. Nine had tumors of the temporal lobe; of this group, 2 were aggressive or assaultive, 2 were suicidal, 1 was both aggressive and suicidal, 1 had episodes of depression, another had episodic uncontrollable fear, and 2 others showed secondary psychotic symptoms and seclusiveness. Patients with tumors of other parts of the limbic system were also described as being hostile, assaultive, and aggressive.

The reason for the eruption of such disturbed behavior is not hard to understand. Under normal conditions, the limbic brain is dominated by and synchronized with the functions of the neocortex. A series of checks and balances exists in both of these parts of the brain, so that the violence associated with the fight-or-flight reactions and governed by the limbic system is kept under control. Damage to the brain structure*—whether by tumors, infection, lack of oxygen, or a blow to the head—upsets the balances between limbic system and neocortex. The perfect synchronization between them that is so necessary for an adequate and reasonable response to environmental stimuli is lost, and so is control over violent inclinations. Sometimes the propensity for violence goes unnoticed, particularly when other symptoms of structural brain disease such as blindness, paralysis, and dementia are so severe that impulsive antisocial acts are impossible or seem irrelevant; nevertheless, the link between structural brain disease and aggressive, assaultive behavior is unquestionably plain.

* The chronic use of brain intoxicants, such as alcohol, associated with vitamin deficiency can also produce altered behavioral states associated with brain degeneration. But since the brain changes are usually not confined to the limbic system, we have not included this complex subject in our monograph. Obviously, individuals who commit violence while acutely intoxicated are behaving, by definition, with a malfunctioning brain.

Epilepsy

Malfunctioning of the brain may result in symptoms that do not involve any apparent change or disease in brain structure. This kind of functional brain disease is also related to uncontrolled violent behavior and certain kinds of epileptic attacks.

What is epilepsy? Epilepsy itself is not a disease. It is a symptom of brain dysfunction and electrical disorganization within the brain. This disorganization is manifested inside the brain as a very noticeable electrical discharge marked by an increase in both amplitude and frequency of the brain waves. The discharges may occur in various parts of the brain (such as the temporal lobe) or in the entire brain. Behavioral symptoms occasionally occur in relation to certain kinds of epileptic spells, such as temporal lobe seizures; but behavioral symptoms also occur between attacks and cannot be distinguished electrically by the inadequate tools that we now use to record brain wave disturbances.

The two kinds of epilepsy related to the brain as a whole are called grand mal and petit mal. Grand mal seizures are initiated usually with a stertorous cry, after which the epileptic person loses consciousness. While he is unconscious, his arm, leg, and trunk muscles may repeatedly contract; he may salivate, bite his tongue, and urinate or defecate. This seizure may last from 30 seconds to 5 minutes; after it is over, he may be confused, tired, and sleepy. A seizure of petit mal epilepsy, which is most often seen in children, is marked by a few seconds' lapse of consciousness, and by staring.

Of the varieties of epilepsy which begin in or are confined to a particular part of the brain, the most important with regard to impulsive or violent behavior is temporal lobe epilepsy; attacks may occur independently or in conjunction with grand mal seizures. A typical attack of temporal lobe epilepsy which includes epileptic foci within the limbic system begins with the sensation of an unusual—often unpleasant—taste or smell (this alerts the neurologist to the fact the "nose brain" is involved), or with a feeling of discomfort in the abdomen, which may include nausea or pain. Sometimes a spell may start with a distorted visual or auditory perception of some object in the environment. The seizure continues with loss or lapse of consciousness, head turning, orienting movements of the eyes, lip smacking, swallowing, and salivation. Some temporal lobe epileptics go through a series of complex and unvarying automatic movements during their seizures, such as buttoning and unbuttoning a shirt, or taking all the clothes out of a drawer and throwing them on the floor.

Emotional disturbances are also present; the epileptic may feel severely depressed or he may be overwhelmed by fear to which he may react by running wildly and aimlessly or by becoming aggressive. Indeed, individuals with temporal lobe seizures or generalized seizures involving the temporal lobe very often have difficulty maintaining control over their behavior. The subjective effects of electrical disturbances in the inner portion of the temporal lobe—that is, in the hippocampus and amygdala—have been reported by people who have had seizures and not lost consciousness. These effects have been exactly duplicated by stimulating the same areas of the brain with surgically implanted electrodes which act as a conduit for electrical or chemical stimulation. In a general way, the reports of individuals experiencing attacks of temporal lobe epilepsy may include:

1. *Perceptual changes*: Most commonly, these are changes in visual perception. The size of an object may vary as if it were receding or approaching. Some individuals report the walls and floor of the room begin to look wavy, or everything looks very small and distant, or quite large. Auditory stimuli are also misperceived. The voices in a room can become very distant; or they may be heard as if everyone were shouting.
2. *Changes in awareness*: Most frequently, these feelings involve depersonalization (loss of a sense of self) and derealization (loss of a sense that the environment is real). Both these misperceptions arouse anxiety and apprehension. The patient may experience *deja vu*, a sudden sense of intense familiarity with a situation, as though the person has already lived through it exactly the same way once before and can predict exactly what is going to happen next. Or the opposite experience (*jamais vu*) may occur when the individual, although in a familiar situation, perceives it as entirely novel and strange. At the same time, in both reactions, the patient, in contrast to a normal person who may have mild sensations of this kind, is usually aware that his feelings are not reasonable. Depersonalization is reported in such phrases as "I am

a disembodied spirit floating along above the clouds, watching my body walk." Derealization is reported as, "It feels as though all the world is on a television screen and I'm watching it," or "All the people on the street seem to be statues except for me."

3. *Changes in thought*: The most striking of these is forced thought—that is, a thought, or word, or sentence intrudes itself on consciousness until it occupies the center of awareness. The thought may be an obscenity, it may be nonsense, it may be a melody. Forced thoughts are also, of course, part of normal experience, but they are apparently much more intense during seizures. Occasionally, the thought may be a complex memory sequence—always remembered in exactly the same way. It may be recalled clearly after the seizure, or remembered vaguely, or even forgotten; generally, though, the temporal lobe epileptic is convinced that he has remembered it before in an identical way. Some temporal lobe epileptics who have been violent report that a persistent and usually unpleasant thought preceded and triggered their uncontrollable violent actions. This is particularly true when the violence is directed toward themselves.
4. *Changes in mood and affect*: The temporal lobe epileptic may suffer fear, anxiety, and terror which are frequently accompanied by some kind of psychic seizure. The anxiety is described as different from the apprehension many epileptics feel just before a seizure occurs. It is felt as isolated, free-floating, and far out of proportion to any external event. The fear may be so intense as to provoke some kind of motor response. Often this takes the form of flight, but if the person is not able or not free to run away, he is apt to react instead with some form of attack behavior. Both fear and rage, however, are minimally related to environmental stimuli.

   Other mood changes include depression that is severe enough to make suicide seem necessary. These feelings of acute despair are quite real, but they seldom have a specific content and usually last only a few minutes. Feelings of pleasure and elation are apparently somewhat rarer; it may be they are seldom reported because they are embarrassing to the individual.
5. *Complex hallucinatory experiences*: During a seizure, quite complex visual, tactile, and auditory hallucinations may

occur. They most often take the form of voices calling the epileptic's name, or voices singing a piece of music. Occasionally, the voices may be so threatening or disturbing that the individual will react with flight or direct attack behavior.

6. *Complex stereotyped automatisms*: These motor movements usually do not last long, but they may involve very complex patterns of behavior tied to the psychic life of temporal lobe epileptics. They may appear purposeful, but they are usually inappropriate; furthermore, they are stereotyped—that is, they recur almost identically during each seizure.

We have described the seizures and manifestations of temporal lobe epilepsy in such detail because these symptoms are very similar to the ones that precede episodes of aggression and poor impulse control in some violent individuals. Such violent episodes are like the seizures of temporal lobe epilepsy in many respects. They may be preceded by changes in perception, by depersonalization, forced thinking, or hallucination; they may include a short period of violent muscular activity followed by exhaustion and relief. However, they are not seizures in the usual sense because there is no loss of consciousness, or even loss of memory for the violent behavior.

The point here, we believe, is that these similar phenomena of episodic violence reflect a functional abnormality in the temporal lobe. This assumption is supported by the observations of many clinicians that people with a structural disease of the temporal lobe are an unusually disturbed group as compared to the general population, and that those with temporal lobe brain wave abnormalities who may or may not have epileptic seizures often share certain behavioral difficulties, including episodes of dyscontrol and violence. Furthermore, although episodes of violence also occur in people with other symptoms of brain disease—such as memory loss, speech difficulties, loss of sight, and grand or petit mal seizures—the coincidence with seizures of temporal lobe epilespsy is frequent. Indeed, most of the violent individuals we have seen and treated surgically suffered from both disorders.

One such person was Mary C., a 48-year-old woman who had had her first grand mal epileptic seizure after the birth of her second child. After five more epileptic attacks, she was successfully treated with the antiseizure medication, Dilantin. Six months later, however, Mary's husband noticed she was having

15- to 20-second lapses of consciousness with staring, head turning, lip smacking, and salivation—that is, she had the symptoms of temporal lobe epilepsy. These seizures occurred at least four or five times a day over the next decade, and like many patients with temporal lobe epilepsy, her condition could not be successfully controlled even with a sophisticated regimen of antiseizure medicines. Over these same 10 years, Mary's personality gradually changed. She had always been bubbly and efferverscent, an unusually happy woman even in the face of adversity. Now she suffered from fits of gloom and surliness, often on days when she had no temporal lobe seizures. Mary was usually not able to remember her seizures, and for many years she denied having any warning that one was coming on; finally, however, she did admit that many of them were preceded first by a feeling of pain or discomfort in her abdomen, then by a deep sensation of anxiety and panic, after which she would lose consciousness and begin her head turning, lip smacking, staring, and salivation.

As the years went by her behavior during a seizure became more elaborate. She would climb the backs of chairs; or she would rush at strangers and throw her arms around them. Her surliness also became more frequent. Worst of all, she insisted on smoking continually, even after she had started a number of small fires during her periods of unconsciouness—fires in which she herself was repeatedly burned. When anyone in her family said anything to her about her constant smoking, she would hit at them with her fists. She also used a broom handle to beat her husband on a dozen different occasions, and once attempted to stab him with a bread knife.

Eventually Mary's violence and her refusal to be reasonable about the dangers inherent in her smoking, as well as her uncontrolled attacks of epilepsy, prompted her physician to seek a surgical opinion. Electrical recordings from her scalp and brain showed typical seizurelike activity, especially in the left amygdala. On the other hand, x-ray films of her brain were not remarkable. But because her clinical state could not be improved by either medicine or psychotherapy, she submitted to a stereotactic surgical destruction of her left amygdala. The initial results of this temporal lobe surgery have been gratifying. She still has seizures but her rages have disappeared. She has set no more fires, and she has become able to function once more as a housewife and mother.

Temporal lobe epilepsy, then, is an important example of a known disease state that is related to violent behavior. This does not mean that we believe that all temporal lobe epileptics are violent, or even have poor impulse control, or that their seizures necessarily include violence. We believe, rather, that temporal lobe disease may cause a number of conditions such as severe recent memory loss, visual field loss, speech difficulties, temporal lobe epilepsy, and poor impulse control—including violent behavior. It is the underlying malfunction in the limbic brain (especially that part in the temporal lobe) that is causally related to poor impulse control and violent behavior. The temporal lobe seizures are only one symptom of such a malfunction but a symptom that no physician can ignore if it occurs in a patient with poor impulse control and violent behavior.

REFERENCES

Aird, R. B., Venturini, A. M., and Spielman, P. M. Antecedents of temporal lobe epilepsy. *Arch. Neurol. 16:*67–73, 1967.

Alpers, B. J. *Personality and Emotional Disorders Associated with Hypothalamic Lesions, in Association in Research in Nervous and Mental Disease.* Baltimore, William & Wilkins, Vol. 20, pp. 725–748, 1940.

Bingley, T. *Mental Symptoms in Temporal Lobe Epilepsy and Temporal Lobe Gliomas.* Stockholm, Kobenhaven, 1958.

Boerhaave, H. *Boerhaave's Aphorisms: Concerning the Knowledge and Cure of Diseases.* (J. Delacoste, trans.) London, W. and J. Innys, 1724.

Bradley, C. Benzedrine and Dexedrine in the treatment of children's behavior disorders. *Pediatrics, 5:*24–36, 1950.

Chao, D., and Davis, S. Convulsive equivalent syndrome of childhood. *J. Pediat. 64:*499–508, 1964.

Davis, E. Explosive and episodic behavior disorder in children as epileptic equivalents *Med. J. Austral. 46:*474–481, 1959.

Delgado, J. M. R., and Hamlin, H. Direct recording of spontaneous and evoked seizures in epileptics. *EEG Neurophysiol. 10:*463–486, 1958.

Delgado, J. M. R. "Comments on Neuropharmacological Studies of EEG and Behavior." In: *EEG and Behavior* (G. H. Glaser, ed.). New York, Basic Books, pp. 284–290, 1963.

Detre, T., and Feldman, R. G. "Behavior Disorder Associated with Seizure States: Pharmacological and Psychosocial Management." In: *EEG and Behavior* (G. H. Glaser, ed.). New York, Basic Books, pp. 366–376, 1963.

Dostoyevsky, F. *The Idiot* (C. Garnett, trans.) New York, Random House, 1935.

Epstein, A. W., and Ervin, F. R. Psychodynamic significance of seizure content in psychomotor eplipsy. *Psychon. Med. 18:*1956.

Ervin, F. R., Epstein, A. W., and King, H. E. Behavior of epileptic and non-epileptic patients with "temporal spikes." *Arch. Neurol. Psychiat. 74:*488–497, 1955.

Ervin, F. R. "Psychiatric Aspects of Epilepsy." In: *Comprehensive Textbook of Psychiatry* (A. Freedman and M. Kaplan, eds.). Baltimore, Williams & Wilkins, 1967.

Faris, A. A. Limbic system infarction. *Neurology 19:*91–96, 1969.

Freeman, F. R., and Nevis, A. H. Temporal lobe sexual seizures. *Neurology 19:*87–90, 1969.

Gastaut, H., and Gastaut, Y. Corrélations électroencéphalographiques et cliniques a propos de 100 cos d'épilepsie dite "psychomotrice" avec foyers sur la region temporales du scalp. *Rev. Oto-neuro-Ophtal. 23:* 257–282, 1951.

Gastaut, H., Terzian, H., Naquet, R., and Luschnat, K. Corrélations entres les "Automatismes" des crises temporales et la phenomenes électroencéphalographiques qui les accompagnent. *Rev. Neurol. 86:* 678–682, 1952.

Gastaut, H. So-called "psychomotor" and "temporal" epilepsies. *Epilepsia 2:*59–76, 1953.

Gastaut, H. Interpretation of the symptoms of "psychomotor" epilepsy in relation to physiologic data on rhinencephalic function. *Epilepsia 3:*84–88, 1954.

Gastaut, H., and Collomb, H. Sexual behavior in psychomotor epileptics. *Ann. Med. Psychol. 112:*657–696, 1954.

Gastaut, H. *The Epilepsies: Their Electro-Clinical Correlates.* Springfield, Ill. Thomas, 1954.

Gastaut, H. Les troubles du comportement alimentaire chez les épileptiques psychomoteurs. *Rev. Neurol. 92:*55–62, 1955.

Gastaut, H., Morin, G., and Lesevre, N. Behavior of psychomotor epileptics between seizures: Disorders of general activity and sociability. *Ann. Med. Psychol. 113:*1–27, 1955.

Gastaut, H., Roger, J., and Giove, C. Olfactory, gustatory and appetite disorders in psychomotor epileptics. *Ann. Med. Psychol. 113:*177–206, 1955.

Gibbs, F. A., Gibbs, E. L., and Lennox, W. G. Epilepsy: A paroxsymal cerebral dysrythmia. *Brain 60:*377–388, 1937.

Gibbs, E. L., Fuster, B., and Gibbs, F. A. Peculiar low temporal localization of sleep-Induced seizure discharges of psychomotor type. *Arch. Neurol. Psychiat. 60:*95–97, 1948.

Gibbs, E. L., Gibbs, F. A., and Fuster, B. Psychomotor epilepsy. *Arch. Neurol. Psychiat. 60:*331–339, 1948.

Gibbs, F. A. Ictal and non-ictal psychiatric disorders in temporal lobe epilepsy. *J. Nerv. Ment. Dis. 113*:522–528, 1951.

Glaser, G. H. (ed.) *EEG and Behavior.* New York, Basic Books, 1963.

Gross, M. D., and Wilson, W. C. Behavior disorders of children with cerebral dysrythmia. *Arch. Gen. Psychiat.* 11:610, 1964.

Henry, C. E. Positive Spike Discharges In the EEG. In: *EEG and Behavior* (G. H. Glaser, ed.). New York, Basic Books, pp. 315–344, 1963.

Hill, D. EEG in episodic psychiatric and psychopathic behavior. *EEG Clin. Neurophysiol. 4*:419, 1952.

Irsigler, F. J. Neurosurgical aspects of brain atrophies. *Acta Neurochirur. 11*:497–512, 1964.

Jackson, J. H. On a particular variety of epilepsy ("intellectual aura"): One case with symptoms of organic brain disease. *Brain 11*:179–207, 1889.

Jackson, J. H., and Beevor, C. E. Case of tumour of the right tempero-sphenoidal lobe bearing on the localization of the sense of smell and on the interpretation of a particular variety of epilepsy. *Brain 12*:346–349, 1890.

Jackson, J. H., and Colman, W. S. Case of epilepsy with tasting movements and "dreamy state"—very small patch of softening in the left unciate gyrus. *Brain 21*:580–590, 1898.

Jackson, J. H., and Stewart, P. Epileptic attacks with a warning of a crude sensation of smell and with the intellectual aura (dreamy state) in a patient who had symptoms pointing to gross organic disease of the right temporo-sphenoidal lobe. *Brain* 22:534–549, 1899.

Jasper, H., and Kershman, J. Electroencephalographic classification of the epilepsies. *Arch. Neurol. Psychiat. 45*:903–943, 1941.

Jasper, J., Pertuiset, B., and Flanigin, H. EEG and cortical electrograms in patients with temporal lobe seizures. *Arch. Neurol. Psychiat.* 65:272–290, 1951.

Keschner, M., Bender, M. B., and Strauss, I. Mental symptoms in cases of tumor of the temporal lobe, *Arch. Neurol. Psychiat. 35*:572–596, 1936.

Keschner, M., Bender, M. B., and Strauss, I. Mental symptoms in cases of subtentorial tumor. *Arch. Neurol. Psychiat. 37*:1–15, 1937.

Killifer, F. A., and Stern, W. E. Chronic effects of hypothalamic injury. *Arch. Neurol.* 22:419–429, 1970.

Kroll, M. "Lyssa (Rabies, Tollwut)." In: *Handbuch der Neurologie* (O. Bumke and O. Foerster, eds.). Berlin, Springer, 1936, pp. 63–88.

Kurland, L. T. The incidence and prevalence of convulsive disorders in a small urban community. *Epilepsia 1*:143–161, 1959.

McLaurin, R. L., and Heimer, F. The syndrome of temporal-lobe contusion. *J. Neurosurg.* 23:296–303, 1965.

MacRae, D. Isolated fear—a temporal lobe aura. *Neurology 4:*497–505, 1954.

Magnus, O., Ponsen, L. and VanRijn, A. J. Temporal lobe epilepsy. *Folia Psychiat. Neerl. 57:*264–297, 1954.

Malamud, N. Psychiatric symptoms and the limbic lobe. *Bull. Los Angeles Neurol. Soc. 22:*131–139, 1957.

Malamud, N. The epileptogenic focus in temporal lobe epilepsy from a pathological standpoint. *Arch. Neurol. 14:*190–195, 1966.

Malamud, N. Psychiatric disorder with intracranial tumors of the limbic system. *Arch. Neurol. 17:*113–123, 1967.

Meyer, A., and Beck, E. The hippocampal formation in temporal lobe epilepsy. *Proc. Roy. Soc. Med. 48:*457–462, 1955.

Meyer-Mickelheit, R. W. Die Dämmerattacken als charakeristischer Anfallstyp der temporalen Epilepsie (psychomotorische Anfalle, Aquivalente, Automatismen). *Nervenarzt. 24:*331–346, 1953.

Mulder, D. W., and Daly, D. Psychiatric symptoms associated with lesions of the temporal lobe. *JAMA 150:*173–176, 1952.

Narabayashi, H., Nagao, R., Saito, Y., Yoshida, M., and Nogabata, M. Stereotaxic amygdalotomy for behavioral disorders. *Arch. Neurol. 9:*1–16, 1963.

Ounstead, C. Hyperkinetic syndrome in epileptic children. *Lancet 2:*303, 1955.

Penfield, W., and Jasper, H. *Epilepsy and the Functional Anatomy of the Brain.* Boston, Little, Brown, 1954.

Reeves, A. G., and Plum, F. Hyperphagia, rage, and dementia accompanying a ventromedial hypothalamic neoplasm. *Arch. Neurol. 20:*616–624, 1969.

Roger, A., and Doniger, M. Correlations electroclinques chez 50 epileptiques internes. *Rev. Neurol. 83:*593–596, 1950.

Sano, K., and Malamud, N. Clinical significance of sclerosis of the cornu Ammonis. *Arch. Neurol. Psychiat. 70:*40–53, 1953.

Sommer, W. Erkrankung des Ammonshorns als aetiologisches Moment der Epilepsie. *Arch. Psychiat. Nervenkr. 10:*631–675, 1880.

Sternlicht, M. Fantasy aggression in delinquent and non-delinquent retardates. *J. Ment. Defic. 70:*819–821, 1966.

Stevens, J. R., Sachdev, K., and Milstein, V. Behavior disorders of children and the electroencephalogram. *Arch. Neurol. 18:*160–177, 1968.

Thomson, A. F., and Walker, A. E. Behavioral alterations following lesions of the medial surface of the temporal lobe. *Folia Psychiat. neerl.* 53:444-452, 1950.

Windle, W. F. Brain damage at birth: Functional and structural modifications with time. *JAMA 206:*1967–1972, 1968.

Chapter 6

The Surgery of Violence

Extreme remedies are very appropriate for extreme diseases.

Hippocrates

Aphorisms—Section I

Most people who have episodes of violence and/or temporal lobe epilepsy can be successfully treated by a judicious mixture of drugs and supportive psychotherapy. The medication used to control episodic violent behavior usually consists of some combination of tranquilizers, psychic energizers, and antiseizure medications, adjusted to individual needs. Sometimes, however, medication and psychotherapy do not work, and in these cases surgical intervention may be helpful.

The traditional surgical treatment of people with severe temporal lobe epilepsy has been lobectomy—the removal of the front part of whichever temporal lobe is diseased. This operation is extremely valuable for many patients with temporal lobe epilepsy; however, it does involve a large incision, extensive removal of bone, and the sacrifice of significant amount of brain cortex, plus other brain tissue that is not diseased. And apart from these drawbacks and risks, lobectomy is not always feasible. It is useless, for example, for persons with many areas of abnormal electrical activity in both their right and left temporal lobes—that is, who suffer from bilateral temporal lobe epilepsy—because although the loss of a single lobe can be sustained, the removal of both temporal lobes has truly disastrous consequences for behavior and memory, and hence should not be done.

It is possible, however, to treat bilateral temporal lobe abnormalities by stereotactic surgery. In this procedure (described in detail below), tiny electrodes are implanted in the brain and used to destroy a very small number of cells in a precisely determined area. As a surgical technique, it has three great advantages over lobectomy: it requires much less of an opening in the surfaces of the brain than lobectomy does; it destroys less than one-tenth as much brain tissue; and once the electrodes have been inserted in the brain, they can be left without harm to the patient until the surgeon is sure which brain cells are firing abnormally and causing the symptoms of seizures and violence.

These cells are identified in two ways: (1) by looking at their spontaneous firing as recorded in electroencephalograms; and (2) by stimulating them with a weak electric current passed into the brain through the electrodes and then observing the resulting behavior. Stereotactic techniques, therefore, offer a unique opportunity to learn about the relationships between brain mechanisms and violent behavior. Among other things, we have already learned that we can both initiate violent behavior and stop it by stimulating different points in the amygdala and hippocampus in patients with temporal lobe disease. These results support the hypothesis that episodic violence may be a symptom of limbic brain disease.

A Case History

We shall use the history of Clara T. to illustrate the value of stereotactic surgery in controlling the violent behavior accompanying bilateral temporal lobe epilepsy. At 62, Clara weighed 86 pounds and had been suffering from epilepsy for 29 years, ever since she had fallen on a patch of ice and sustained such a severe head injury that she had been unconscious for several days. She subsequently began to have both grand mal and temporal lobe epileptic seizures. Her temporal lobe seizures were ushered in by a feeling of nausea deep in the pit of her stomach and a sensation of impending doom. She did not move much during her spells; she simply stared blankly and smacked her lips for periods of 1 to 3 minutes. The frequency of her temporal lobe seizures gradually increased despite a variety of antiseizure medicines. About 10 years ago an extensive neurological evaluation, including both brain wave examination and special x-ray films of the brain, revealed that abnormalities in her left temporal lobe were responsible. Therefore, her left anterior temporal lobe was removed, after which the tempo of her seizures decreased for about 4 months, and then started to pick up again. At this point, Clara's memory began to fail. Her behavior became unpredictable and she physically assaulted almost anybody who came near her. She used her teeth and nails on an infirm mother-in-law, on delivery boys who came to her house with groceries or newspapers, and on her husband. Eventually, these violent assaults led to her being readmitted to our neurosurgical service 4 years after her lobectomy.

Because of Clara's history of violence, she was admitted to a private room, and all the precautions usual in treating epileptic patients were taken in caring for her. Late one evening she cried out quite suddenly. The nurse on duty thought Clara was about to have an epileptic seizure, and therefore came over to her carrying a padded tongue blade to insert between Clara's teeth to prevent involuntary tongue biting. Clara interpreted the nurses' advance with the tongue blade as an attack, and immediately launched a counterassault. A call for help brought three other nurses and two male orderlies, and all six were not able to get this 86-pound elderly woman back in bed until 45 minutes later. Even then two of them needed medical attention to repair the wounds inflicted by her teeth and nails. Thereafter, Clara was kept in a locked psychiatric ward until she was due for surgery.

Medical and neurological tests showed that Clara had extensive disease in her remaining temporal lobe. As we have already mentioned, removal of her second temporal lobe was out of the question because it would have had such disastrous effects on behavior and memory; consequently, we used stereotactic surgery instead. We were primarily operating to control her epileptic seizures, but we also wanted to reduce or eliminate her rage behavior.

The stages in the operative procedure are shown in Figures 8 through 14. First, a small opening is made in the scalp, skull, and the membrane covering the brain (the dura); second, a

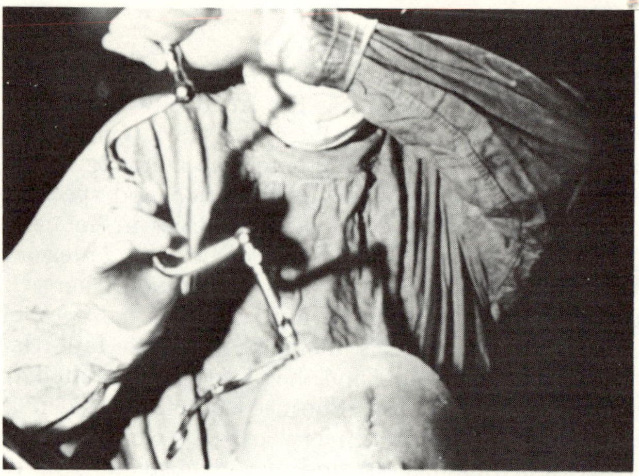

a

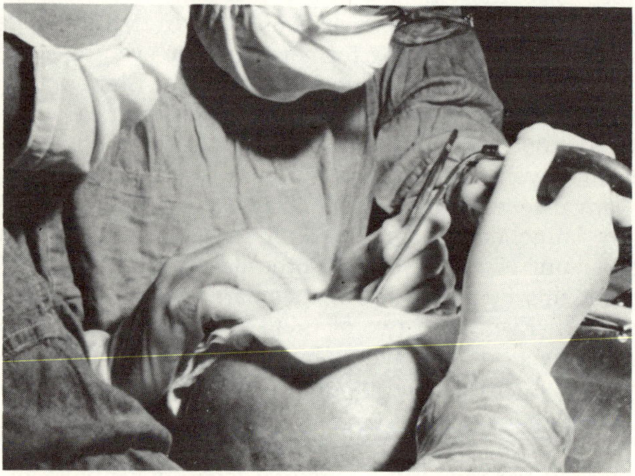

b

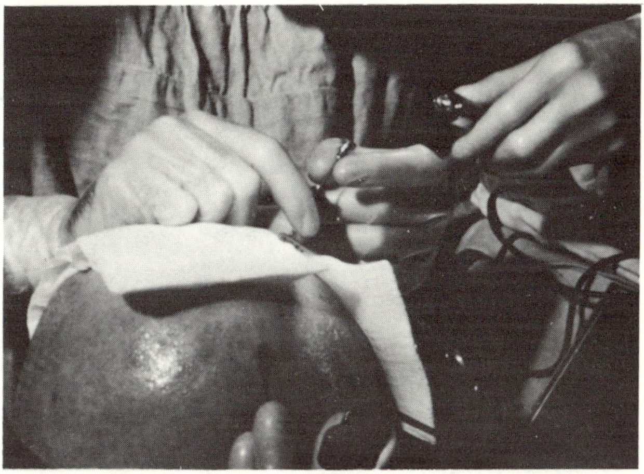

c

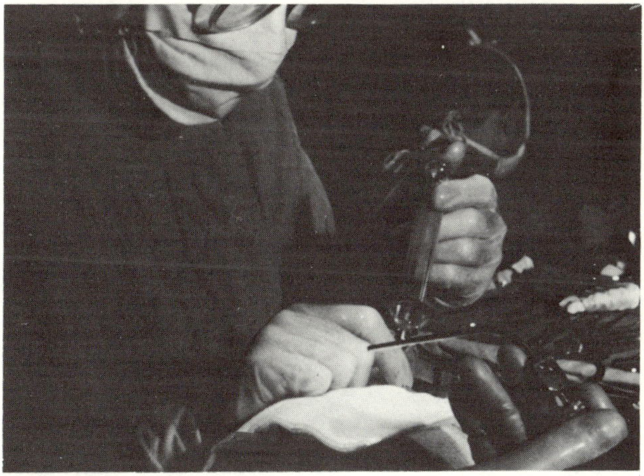

d

FIG. 8. Stereotactic surgery: Stage 1. Stereotactic surgical procedure employs the following sequence. (*a*) Small opening is made in the skull with surgical drill. (*b*) Delicate membrane surrounding brain is incised. (*c*) Slender, hollow, blunt-tipped needle is inserted through brain surface into fluid-filled cavity within brain (ventricle). (*d*) Radiopaque solution is injected into ventricle to opacify important landmarks—used in subsequent x-rays to identify target areas within brain.

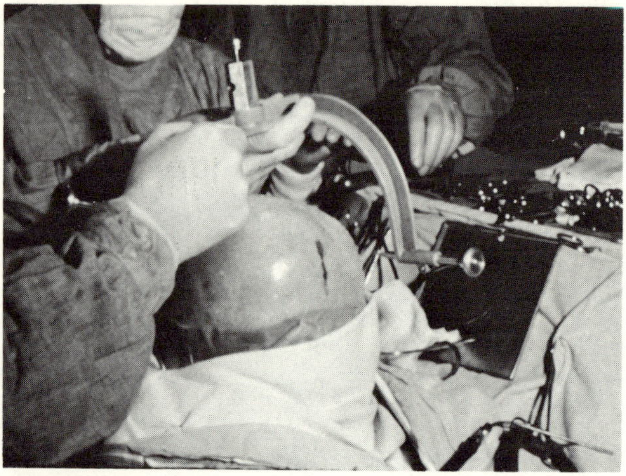

a

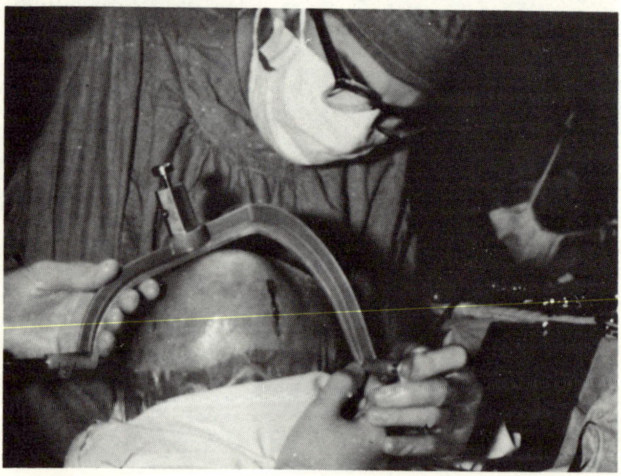

b

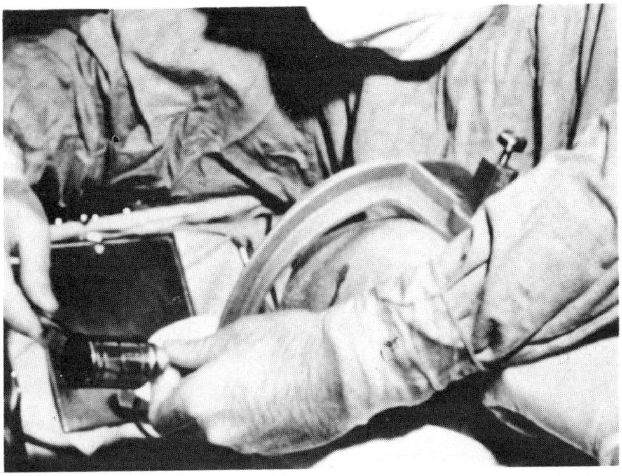

c

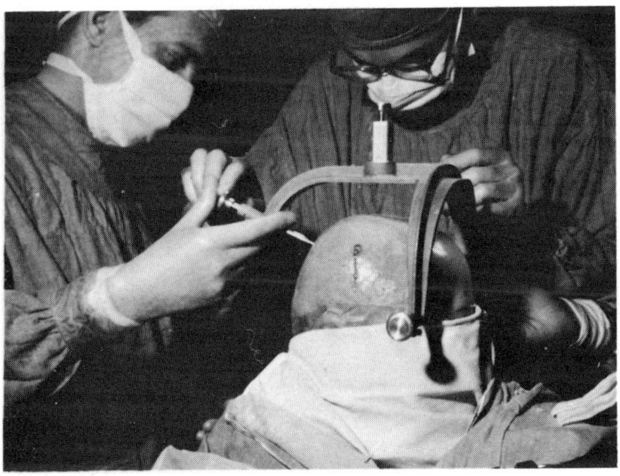

d

FIG. 9. Stereotactic surgery: Stage 2. Special instrument used to guide electrode to deep target structures is called stereotactic machine. Here it is fixed to skull by means of three sharp metal pins.

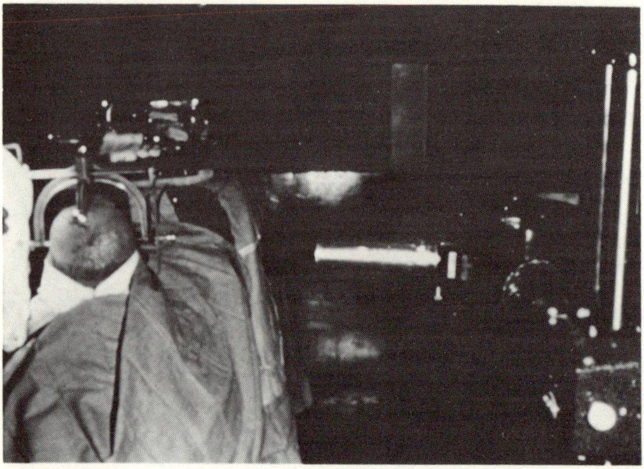

a

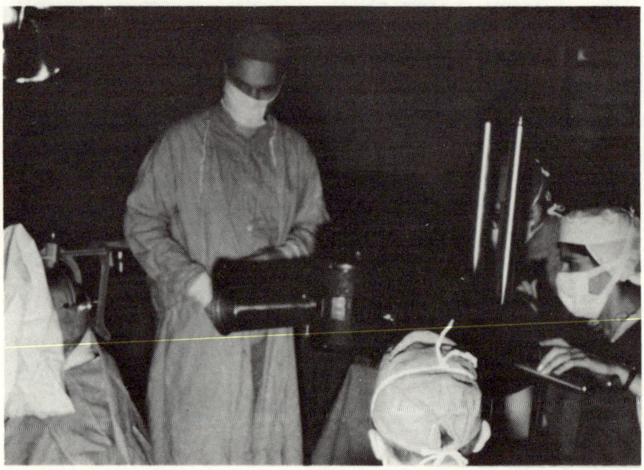

b

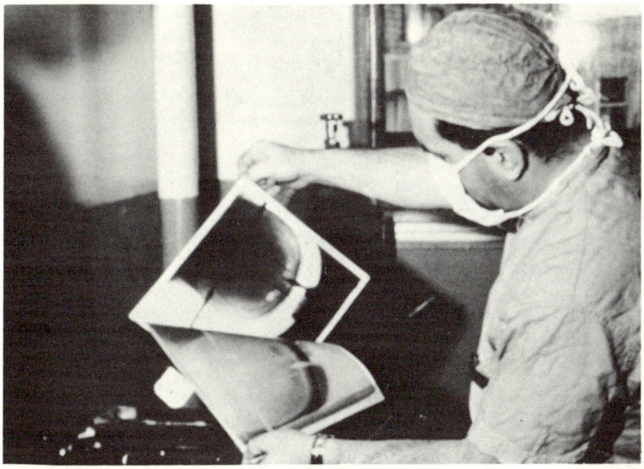

c

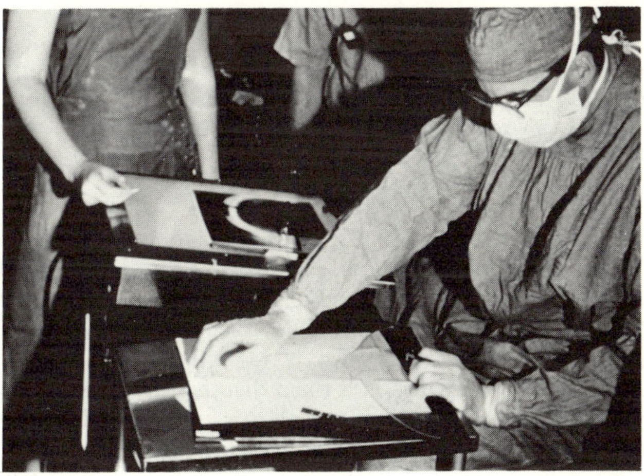

d

FIG. 10. Stereotactic surgery: Stage 3. (*a*) and (*b*) Lead grids are fixed to stereotactic machine and x-ray films are taken with a fixed distance between x-ray tube and x-ray plate or *cassette*. (*c*) Rapid-developing Polaroid x-ray film is used to visualize important brain landmarks. (*d*) Plotting chart is used to translate measurements from x-ray to settings for stereotactic machine.

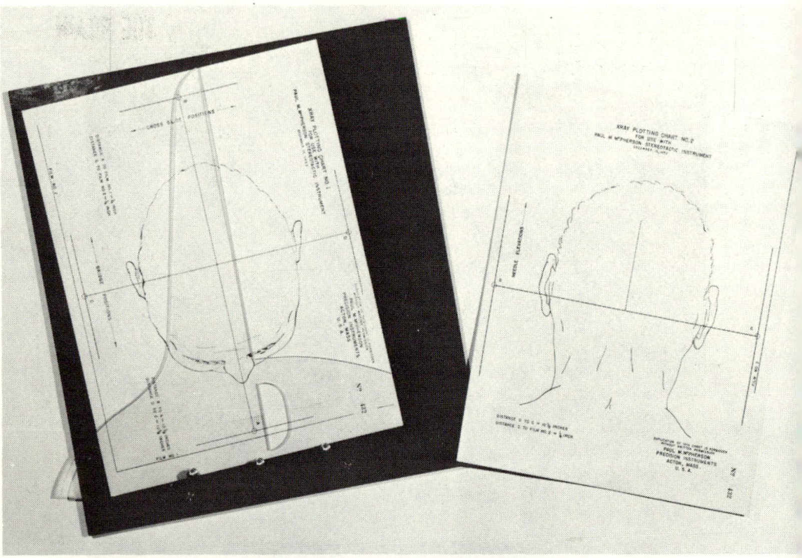

FIG. 11. Stereotactic surgery: Stage 4. This shows our plotting charts in more detail. They contain crossing lines that are geometrically identical to lead cross hairs of stereotactic machine. Straight edge of plastic rule can reduplicate any central x-ray beam. The two charts together can identify any point on the x-ray that we can see with an error of less than 0.5 mm.

blunt needle is inserted into the fluid-filled space within the brain (the ventricle), and a small quantity of radiopaque dye is instilled through the needle (Fig. 8). Next, a guiding instrument, the stereotactic machine, is fixed to the skull at three points (Fig. 9). An x-ray film is taken, the x-ray equipment being set up so that there is a fixed distance between the source of the x-ray beam and the x-ray plate (Fig. 10). The x-ray film is read to measure the distance between the brain structures that were visualized by the opaque material (such as the temporal horn of the ventricle) and the target (such as the amygdala), which cannot be visualized on x-ray examination. This gives a preliminary setting for our stereotactic instrument, enabling us to place our electrode in the area of the target. This is accomplished with the aid of a plotting chart (see Fig. 11) which is used to translate measurements from the x-ray to settings on the stereotactic machine. These measurements are reproduced on a "phantom" (Fig. 12), an exact duplicate of the stereotactic

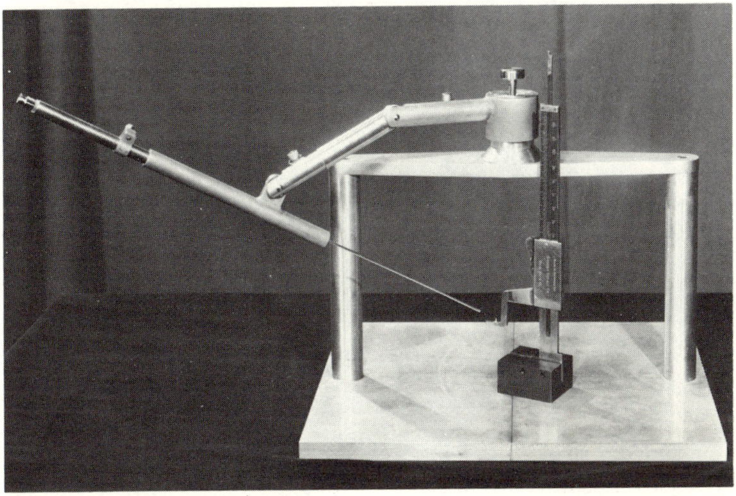

FIG. 12. Stereotactic surgery: Stage 5. This phantom stereotactic machine is used to position our stereotactic electrode and lock it on the target before it is placed in real stereotactic machine on patient's head. Base of phantom is identical to our plotting charts. Lever arm and collar of phantom are in identical positions as compared to same equipment on real stereotactic machine.

machine, to complete the translation from x-ray setting to stereotactic measurements. When the electrode has reached the target on the phantom (Fig. 13), all moving parts of the stereotactic machine are locked into place. Then the stereotactic guide is lifted from the phantom and applied to the stereotactic machine fitted to the patient's head. The electrode is then inserted through the skull opening, dura, and brain into the target area. Final adjustments of our electrode—increasing our precision, and confirming our placement—are made with the aid of physiological tools such as the recording of deep brain potentials, noting the effects of stimulation, or the production of temporary blockade of neural activity in the target area with a slight elevation or depression of the temperature around the electrode tip. Finally, the electrode is locked into position, if it is to be left in place (Fig. 14), and the tail of the electrode is brought out at a distant point through the scalp.

We implanted four multilead electrodes in Clara's brain: two in the right temporal lobe and two in what remained of her left temporal lobe after the lobectomy (Fig. 15).

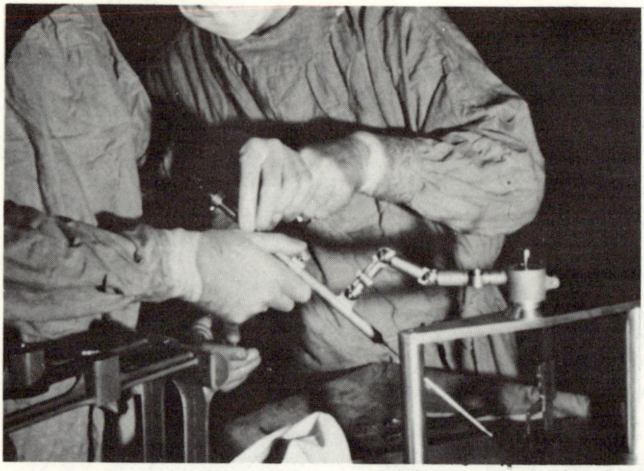

a

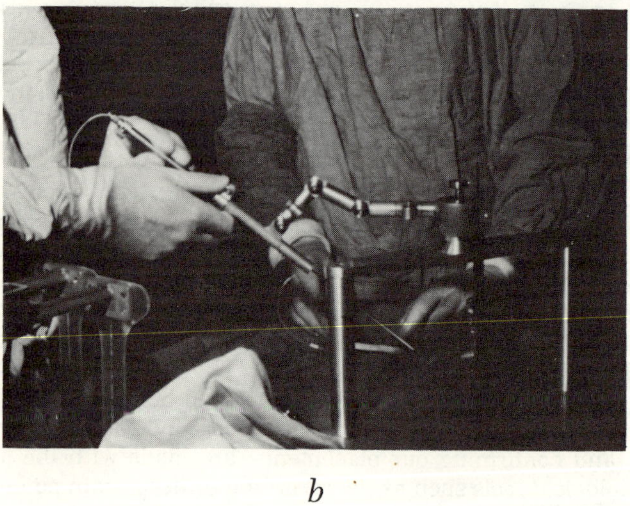

b

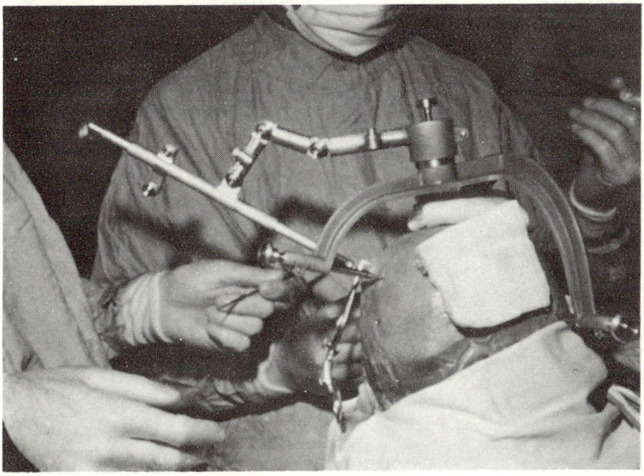

c

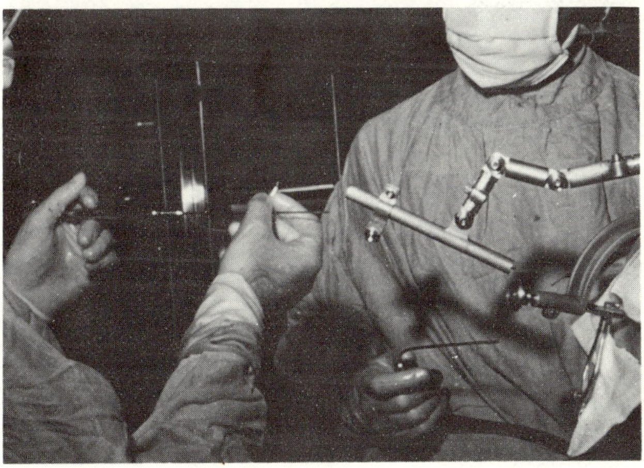

d

FIG. 13. Stereotactic surgery: Stage 6. (*a*) and (*b*) Plotting chart settings of target are set up on phantom and collar and lever arm are locked into place. (*c*) Collar and lever arm are transferred to stereotactic machine. (*d*) Electrode is about to be inserted into lever arm holder.

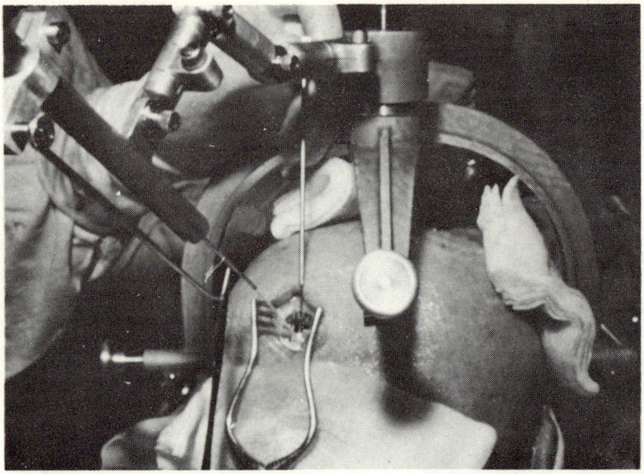

a

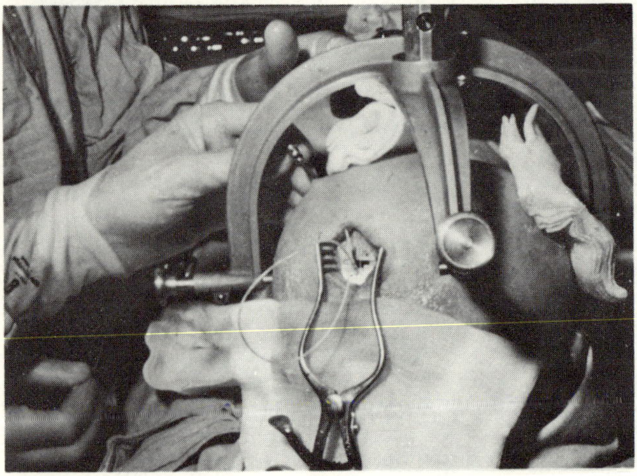

b

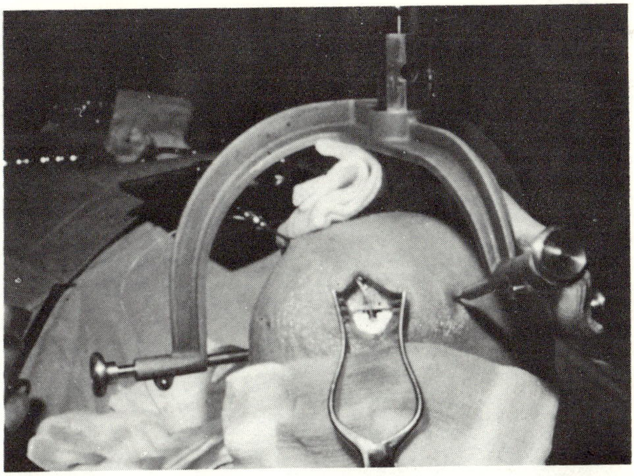

c

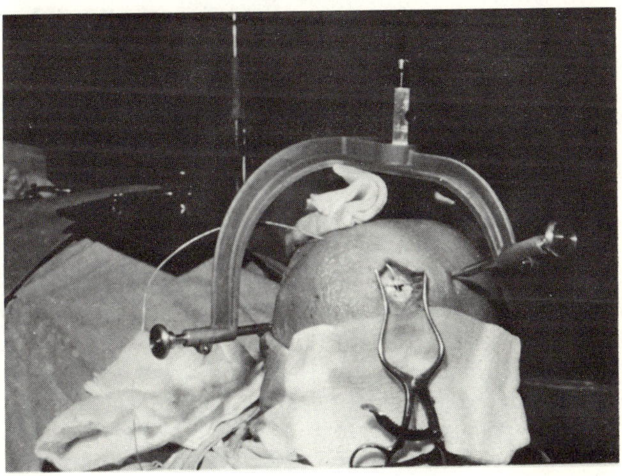

d

FIG. 14. Stereotactic surgery: Stage 7. (*a*) Electrode has been inserted into region of brain target (final adjustments having been aided by physiological recordings). As electrode is going to remain in position for several weeks, it is locked into position by metal plug or cemented in position. (*b*) Tail of electrode is brought out of the scalp through needle which punctures scalp 6 cm. distant from wound. (*c*) Electrode is fed into needle. (*d*) Needle is removed, leaving tail of electrode emerging from small scalp opening 6 cm. from wound.

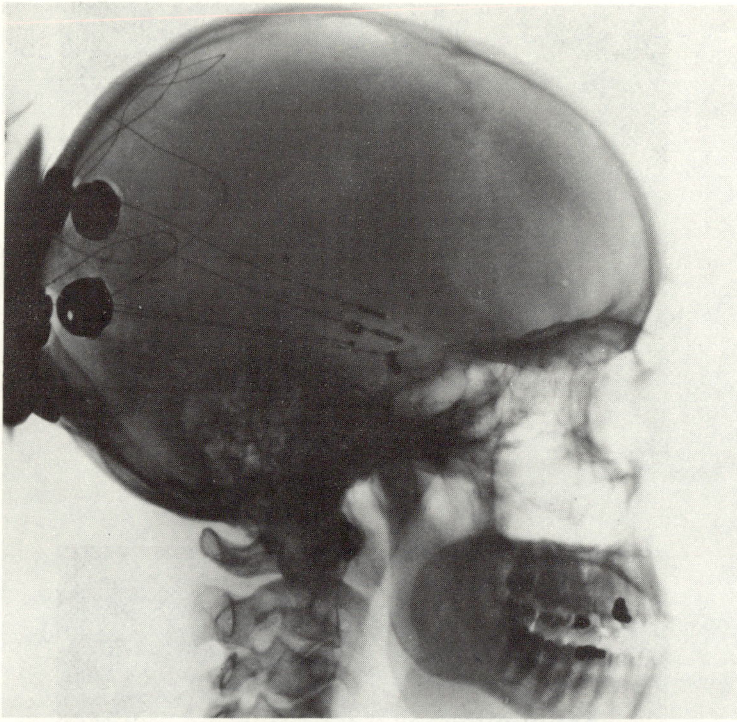

FIG. 15. X-ray film shows electrodes in amygdala similar to those of patient Clara T. on the side opposite the temporal lobectomy.

When Clara had recovered from her operation, we recorded the electrical brain activity next to the forty exposed electrode points (twenty in each temporal lobe. The brain waves from the depth electrode in her right temporal lobe showed a clear-cut area of abnormal electrical activity in and around the amygdala. Furthermore, when we used weak electrical currents to stimulate this same area of the brain, she reacted by having one of her seizures. These findings did not change over a period of 6 weeks. At that time, we began slowly to inactivate the abnormal region we had identified in her right amygdala. We did this by applying radiofrequency current through the appropriate electrode point. The current generates a temperature of 65°C, and this heat is enough to destroy a very limited number of brain cells around the tip of the electrode.

We waited for another month, then withdrew the electrodes.

During this time, Clara had no episodes of rage. Her epileptic seizures continued; however, their character had changed—they consisted of short lapses of consciousness without any abdominal discomfort or chewing movements.

We have watched Clara's progress for nearly 6 years. The frequency of her epileptic seizures has diminished and her rages and unprovoked assaults have not recurred at all. She has been able to resume a more normal life, both in the community and at home. We did not achieve our goal of controlling her epileptic seizures; nonetheless, we did stop her rage attacks and the results of the operation are thus gratifying.

Clara's case is important for several reasons. First it shows that surgical treatment can be used effectively to stop abnormal attacks of rage. Secondly, it demonstrates the separation of rage and epilepsy. The operation had a striking effect on the former even though it had but a slight effect on the latter. Patients with temporal lobe epilepsy have been successfully treated by stereotactic surgery, but we should like to concentrate in this monograph on the treatment of rage.

Other Experience

The use of stereotactic destruction of the amygdala as a clinical tool for the control of violent behavior rather than for the management of temporal lobe epilepsy alone was pioneered by Narabayashi of Japan. In 1965, he reported on 98 patients on whom he had operated for the treatment of episodic destructive episodes accompanying various kinds of diffuse brain disease. All of his patients were mentally defective to begin with. Thirteen were adults, of whom 11 had epilepsy. Four epileptics were dramatically improved. Three were improved but relapsed in 6 to 12 months and six were not improved. Of 27 mentally defective assaultive children (including 19 epileptics), 14 showed dramatic improvement; 9 were significantly improved and no one was made worse in this series.

Professor Heimberger of the University of Indiana performed stereotactic destructions in the amygdala on 25 severely epileptic patients. Eight of these operations were done on both sides—that is, on both temporal lobes. All of these patients had aggressive behavior or depression. The characteristic symptoms of the patients in this group included not only depression but also hyperactivity, hostility, aggressiveness, and hypersexuality. The behavioral abnormality was eliminated completely in 7 of 20 patients and was markedly improved in many of the others. Convulsions were eliminated in 4 of 21 patients and improved in 12. Overall improvement was noted in 23 of the 25 patients operated on, and 2 of the 12 patients who had been committed to a state institution were released at the completion of the postoperative period.

The treatment of violent behavior by bilateral amygdala destruction has not only been carried out by our own group in Boston but also by surgeons in Japan, India, Mexico, France, and Denmark. Professor Vaernet of Copenhagen has done amygdalotomies in 45 patients with psychomotor epilepsy (i.e., temporal lobe epilepsy); some of these patients had engaged in dangerous behavior, some had not. These lesions were made bilaterally in 9 of these patients, only 1 of whom has shown persistent worsening of any aspect of his behavior. This change consists of a loss of initiative, with a lower score on intelligence tests, and is also associated with the finding of a dilated lateral ventricle 8 months after the second operation. Of the 9 patients, 4 had adequate control of their psychomotor seizures after operation. Two of these 4 patients were violent before operation: 1 of the 2 is strikingly and the other is moderately improved after amygdalotomy. Of the 5 patients with continuing psychomotor seizures, 3 were also violent and all 3 showed a striking improvement in this aspect of their behavior. Another large series of "psychotic" patients with violent behavior were reported separately with a larger proportion of patients relieved of their violent symptoms but with no change in their other manifestations of psychotic behavior.

Sano (and other surgeons in Japan) bypass the amygdala and go directly to the hypothalamus with their stereotactic surgical probe. They place tiny destructive lesions in the posterior portion of the hypothalamus for the control of assaultive behavior in brain-damaged children. They have labeled this technique "sedative surgery." They believe that this method has been more effective than amygdala destruction in treating the symptoms manifested by this difficult group of patients. More recently, stereotactic lesions in the medial thalamus have also proved to be effective in returning patients with abnormal assaultive behavior to a normal status. It is of interest that some of the earliest work done with the stereotactic machine by

Spiegel and Wycis included lesions in the thalamus in disturbed schizophrenic patients.

In summary, then, there is a significant and growing body of clinical and especially surgical evidence to indicate that the production of small focal areas of destruction in parts of the limbic brain will often eliminate dangerous behavior in assaultive or violent patients. That this therapeutic effect is not always obtained may be explained in some patients by the presence of brain disease in central structures (e.g., the midbrain) that are not controlled directly by the amygdala. In addition, there are competing systems in the limbic brain that both initiate and stop violent behavior. As surgeons we are only beginning to recognize the subtleties of this complex region. It is our expectation that a better understanding of the structure and function of the limbic brain will help us perfect our treatment.

In this chapter we have concentrated on the surgical treatment of violence rather than on the medical and psychological methods. We have not done this to downgrade the importance of the latter. In the context of this monograph, however, we are attempting to relate violent behavior to brain function and specifically to the activity of the limbic brain. And although violent behavior and suicidal attempts can often be controlled by a judicious combination of tranquilizers, anticonvulsants, psychic energizers, and psychotherapy, too little is known about the modes of action of these agents, at present, to add cogent factual data to our thesis.

REFERENCES

Andy, O. Thalamotomy in Hyperactive and Aggressive Behavior. Presented before the International Society for Research in Stereoencephalotomy, New York, September 27, 1969.

Aronow, S. The use of radiofrequency power in making lesions in the brain. *J. Neurosurg. 17:*431–438, 1960.

Bailey, P., and Stein, S. U. "A Stereotaxic Instrument for Use on the Human Brain." In: *Studies in Medicine.* Springfield, Ill., Thomas, pp. 40–49, 1951.

Brodkey, J. S., Miyazaki, Y., Ervin, F. R., and Mark, V. H. Reversible heat lesion with radiofrequency current: A method of stereotactic localization. *J. Neurosurg. 21:*49–53, 1964.

Crandall, P. H., Walter, R. D., and Rand, R. W. Clinical application of studies on stereotactically implanted electrodes in temporal lobe epilepsy. *J. Neurosurg. 20:*827–840, 1963.

Delgado, J. M. R., Hamlin, H., and Chapman, W. P. Technique of intracerebral electrode placement for recording and stimulation and its possible therapeutic value in psychotic patients. *Confin. Neurol. 12:*315–319, 1952.

Delgado, J. M. R., and Hamlin, H. Intracerebral recording of the frontal lobes in psychotic and non-psychotic patients. *EEG Clin. Neurophysiol. 6:*703, 1954.

Delgado, J. M. R. Use of intracerebral electrodes in human patients. *EEG Clin. Neurophysiol. 8:*528–530, 1956.

Ervin, F. R., and Mark, V. H. Stereotactic thalamotomy in the human: Part II. Physiological observations on the human thalamus. *Arch. Neurol. 3:*368–380, 1960.

Ervin, F. R. and Mark, V. H. Studies on the human thalamus: IV. Evoked responses. *Ann. NY Acad. Sci. 112:*81–93, 1964.

Ervin, F. R., and Belsasso, G. "Stereotactic Treatment of Temporal Lobe Epilepsy: Neurophysiologic and Behavioral Observations." In: *Homana an el XXV Anicersario Profesional,* Mexico, 1964, pp. 55–74.

Ervin, F. R., Brown, C. E., and Mark, V. H. Striatal influence on facial pain. *Confin. Neurol. 27:*75–86, 1966.

Falconer, M. A., Meyer, A., Hill, D., Mitchell, W., and Pond, D. A. Treatment of temporal-lobe epilepsy by temporal lobectomy. *Lancet 268:*827–835, 1955.

Falconer, M. A., and Davis, C. T. Surgical treatment of drug-resistant epilepsy due to mesial temporal sclerosis. *Arch. Neurol. 19:*353–361, 1968.

Feindel, W., and Penfield, W. Localization of discharge in temporal lobe automatism. *Arch. Neurol. Psychiat. 72:*605–630, 1954.

Hassler, R., and Riechert, T. Uben einen Fall von doppelseitiger Fornicotomie bei sogenannter temporaler Epilepsie. *Acta Neurochir. 5:*330–340, 1957.

Hassler, R., and Riechert, T. Klinische und anatomische Befunde bei stereotaktischen Schmerzoperationen im Thalamus. *Arch. Psych. Nervenkr. 200:*93–122, 1959.

Hassler, G. "Anatomy of the Thalamus." In: *Introduction to Stereotaxis with an Atlas of the Human Brain, Vol. I* (G. Schaltenbrand and P. Bailey, eds.). New York, Grune & Stratton, pp. 230–290, 1959.

Heath, R. G., and Mickle, W. A. "Evaluation of Seven Years' Experience with Depth Electrode Studies in Human patients." In: *Electrical Studies on the Unanesthetized Brain* (E. R. Ramey and D. S. O'Doherty, eds.). New York, Hoeber, 1960.

Heath, R. G. "Closing Remarks, with Commentary on Depth Electroencephalography in Epilepsy and Schizophrenia." In: *EEG and Behavior* (G. H. Glaser, ed.). New York, Basic Books, pp. 377–393, 1963.

Heimberger, R. R. Stereotaxic amygdalotomy. *JAMA 198:*741–745, 1966.

Horsley, V., and Clarke, R. H. Structure and function of cerebellum examined by a new method. *Brain 31:*45–124, 1908.

Jasper, H., and Rasmussen, T. Studies of clinical and electrical responses to deep temporal stimulation in men with some considerations of functional anatomy. *Res. Nerv. Ment. Dis. Proc., 36:*316–334, 1958.

Leksell, L. A stereotaxic apparatus for intracerebral surgery. *Acta. Chir. Scand. 99:*229–233, 1950.

Mark, V. H., McPherson, P. M., and Sweet, W. H. A new method for correcting distortion in cranial roentgenograms: With special reference to a new human stereotactic instrument. *Amer. J. Roentg. 71:*435–444, 1954.

Mark, V. H., Ervin, F. R., and Hackett, T. P. Clinical aspects of stereotactic thalamotomy in the human: Part I. The treatment of chronic severe pain. *Arch. Neurol. 3:*351–367, 1960.

Mark, V. H., Sweet, W. H., and McPherson, P. M. Stereotactic surgery: A note on instrumentation. *J. Neurol. Neurosurg. Psychiat. 25:*86–89, 1962.

Mark, V. H., Ervin, F. R., and Yakovlev, P. I. Stereotactic thalamotomy: III. The verification of anatomical lesion sites in the human thalamus. *Arch. Neurol. 8:*528–538, 1963.

Mark, V. H., and Ervin, F. R. "Relief of Pain by Stereotactic Surgery." In: *Pain and the Neurosurgeon: A Forty Year Experience.* J. C. White and W. H. Sweet, eds.). Springfield, Ill., Thomas, pp. 834–887, 1969.

Mark, V. H., Ervin, F. R., and Sweet, W. H. The Effect of Amygdalotomy on Violent Behavior in Patients with Temporal Lobe Epilepsy. Presented before the Society of Neurological Surgeons. Boston, Mass., April, 1970.

Narabayashi, H. Stereoencephalotomy in Japan. *Confin. Neurol. 24:* 314–320, 1964.

Narabayashi, H. Stereotaxic amygdalotomy for behavioral and emotional disorders. *Brain Nerve (Japan) 16:*800–804, 1964.

Narabayashi, H., and Uno, M. Long range results of stereotaxic amygdalotomy for behavioral disorders. *Confin. Neurol. 27:*168–171, 1966.

Poblete, M., Stereotaxic Thalamotomy (lamella medialis) in aggressive psychiatric patients. Presented before the International Society for Research in Stereoencephalotomy. New York, September 27, 1969.

Ramamurthi, B., and Balasubramanian, V. Stereotaxic amygdalectomy for behavior disorder. Read by title before the International Society for Research in Stereoencephalotomy. New York, September 27, 1969.

Ramey, E. R., and O'Doherty, D. S. (eds.) Electrical Studies on the Unanesthetized Brain. New York, Hoeber, 1960.

Riechert, R., and Mundinger, F. Beschreibung und Anwendung eines Zielgerates fur stereotakt. Hirnoperationen. *Act. Neurochirurg. (Suppl.) 3:*308–337. 1955.

Sano, K., Yoshioka, M., Ogashiwa, M., Ishijima, B., and Ohye, C. Posteromedial hypothalamotomy in the treatment of aggressive behavior. *Confin. Neurol.* 27:164–167, 1966.

Schaltenbrand, G., and Bailey, P. *Introduction to Stereotaxis with an Atlas of the Human Brain, 3 vols.* New York, Grune & Stratton, 1959.

Schunk, H., and Mark, V. H. "Stereotactic Operations with Particular Consideration of Radiographic Problems." In: *Clinical Neuroradiology* (K. Decker, ed. Amer. edition; W. H. Shehadi, Trans.). New York, McGraw-Hill, pp. 421–439, 1966.

Schwab, R., Sweet, W. H., Mark, V. H., Kjellberg, R. N. and Ervin, F. R. Treatment of intractable temporal lobe epilepsy by stereotactic amygdala lesions. *Trans. Amer. Neurol. Ass. 90:*12–19, 1965.

Spiegel, E. A., Wycis, H. T., Marks, M. and Lee, A. J. Stereotaxis apparatus for operations on the human brain. *Science 106:*349–350, 1947.

Spiegel, E. A., Wycis, H. T., Freed, H., and Lee, A. J. Stereoencephalotomy. *Proc. Soc. Exp. Biol. Med. 69:*175–177, 1948.

Spiegel, E. Wycis, H. T., and Thur, C. The stereoencephalotome. *J. Neursurg. 8:*452–453, 1951.

Spiegel, E. A., and Wycis, H. T. "Stereoencephalotomy (Thalamotomy and Related Procedures): Part I." In: *Methods and Stereotaxis Atlas of the Human Brain.* New York, Grune & Stratton, 1952.

Spiegel, E. A., and Wycis, H. T. Stereoencephalotomy: Part II. In: *Clinical and Physiological Applications.* New York, Grune & Stratton, 1962.

Sweet, W. H., Mark, V. H., and Hamlin, H. Radiofrequency lesions in the central nervous system of man and cat: Including case reports of eight bulbar pain-tract interruptions. *J. Neurosurg. 17:*213–225, 1960.

Talairach, J., Hecaen, H., David, M., Monnier, M., and Ajuriaguerra, J. Recherches sur la coagulation therapeutique des structures souscorticales chez l'homme. *Rev. Neurol. 81:*4–24, 1949.

Talairach, J. Chirurgie stereotaxique du thalamus (Bases anatomique et techniques; Indiations et resultats therapeutiques). *Cong. Latino-Amer. VI, Montevideo,* 865–925, 1955.

Talairach, J., David, M., Tournoux, P., Corredor, H. and Kvasina, T. *Atlas d'Anatomie Stereotaxique.* Paris, Masson, 1957.

Talairach, J., David, M., and Tournoux, P. L'exploration Chirurgicale Stéréotaxique du Lobe Temporale dans L'épilepsie Temporale: Repérage Anatomique et Technique Chirurgicale. Paris, Masson, 1958.

Turner, E. New approach to unilateral and bilateral lobotomies for psychomotor epilepsy. *J. Neurol. Neurosurg. Psychiat.* 26:284–299, 1963.

Umbach, W., and Riechert, T. Stereotactic coagulation of the fornix for temporal epilepsy. *Proc. 1st Int. Congr. Neurol. Sci.* 3:565–578, 1959.

Vaernet, K. On amygdalotomy—personal communication to William H. Sweet, 1969.

Walker, A. E. Stereotaxic methods for the study of subcortical activity in epilepsy. *Confin. Neurol.* 22:217–222, 1962.

Wycis, H. T., Baird, H. W., III, and Spiegel, E. A. Long range results following pallidotomy and pallidoamygdalotomy in certain types of convulsive disorders. *Confin. Neurol.* 27:114–120, 1960.

Yakovlev, P. I., Kury, G., Abramowicz, A., and Chapman, W. P. Stereotactic coordinates of deep cerebral structures in man. Personal communication to V. H. Mark, 1959.

Chapter 7

Brain Triggers for Violence

> ***Arts and sciences are not cast in a mold, but are formed and perfected by degrees, by often handling and polishing, as bears leisurely lick their cubs into form.***
>
> ***Montaigne***
>
> **Essays—Book II, Chapter 12**

The changes in perception, mood, and thought that immediately precede the staring, the head turning, and the lip smacking manifestations of temporal epileptic seizures also occur in individuals with temporal lobe disease who do not have epileptic attacks. In these individuals the changes may mark the beginning of an episode of abnormal behavior, including violence or assault. We have found it is possible to reproduce all these signs of temporal lobe disease, including the violence, by passing weak electrical currents through the tip of a probe implanted in the amygdala. Furthermore, by varying the characteristics of the stimulating current, and by changing the target area of the brain being stimulated, we have found we can both initiate and stop assaultive behavior. The target areas that enable us to accomplish this are in close proximity to one another in the amygdala.

The first time we were able to demonstrate that systems in the limbic brain both start and stop attack behavior was with patient Thomas R. He was a brillant 34-year-old engineer with several important patents to his credit. Despite his muscular physique it was difficult to believe he was capable of an act of violence when he was not enraged, for his manner was quiet and reserved, and he was both courteous and sympathetic.

His history of illness started 14 years earlier, when he had been in the army and stationed in an isolated outpost. At that time, Thomas suffered the rupture of a peptic ulcer, and went into deep shock. By the time he was flown to a hospital, he had had so prolonged a drop in his blood pressure, with resulting brain anemia, that his brain was severely damaged. His ulcer was successfully repaired, but he remained in a coma for 3 days after the operation.

When Thomas was discharged from the army, he educated himself as an engineer. He was an extremely talented, inventive man, but his behavior at times was unpredictable and even frankly psychotic. He was seen and treated by psychiatrists over a period of 7 years with no effect on his destructive outbursts of violence.

Thomas's chief problem was his violent rage; this was sometimes directed at his co-workers and friends, but it was mostly expressed toward his wife and children. He was very paranoid, and harbored grudges which eventually produced an explosion of anger. He often felt that people were gratuitously insulting to him; when he was driving to work in the morning, for instance, and another car cut in front of him, he would take it as a personal affront. Nor was he willing to let any such insult go unpunished. He would speed after the other driver, weaving in and out of traffic, threatening pedestrians, and going through stop signs until he finally caught up to the driver and forced him to the side of the road. If the other driver were a man, Thomas would then hit him; if it were a woman he would insult her.

The assaults against his wife characteristically began after a complaint of severe abdominal or facial pain. During the ensuing conversation, he would seize upon some innocuous remark and interpret it as an insult. At first, he would try to ignore what she had said, but could not help brooding; and the more he thought about it, the surer he felt that his wife no longer loved him and was "carrying on with a neighbor." Eventually he would reproach his wife for these faults, and she would hotly deny them. Her denials were enough to set him off into a frenzy of violence. He would sometimes pick his wife up and throw her against the wall; he did this to her even when she was pregnant. He did the same thing to his children. These periods of rage usually lasted for 5 to 6 minutes, after which he would be overcome with remorse and grief and sob as uncontrollably as he had raged. He would then go to sleep for a half-hour or so and wake up feeling refreshed and eager to work.

Thomas was referred to our hospital by his psychiatrist who had observed the patient as he was having a typical temporal lobe seizure, with staring, lip smacking, and salivation. In the hospital he was found to have periods of confusion and a number of psychotic delusions and hallucinations. His grades on tests for memory were significantly lower than those in tests for arithmetic, word comprehension, and word association. A brain wave examination disclosed epileptic electrical activity in both temporal regions, and special x-ray examination of the brain revealed that one ventricle was larger than the other, with some evidence of brain shrinkage.

Over a period of 7 months, we tried many combinations of antiseizure medicines, tranquilizers, and psychic energizers. Unfortunately, none of these drugs helped, and since both temporal lobes were involved we decided to treat his illness with stereotactic surgery. Arrays of electrodes implanted into each temporal lobe confirmed that electrical discharges typical of epileptic seizures occurred in both the right and the left temporal lobes. Both strands of electrodes in each temporal lobe ended in the nucleus amygdala. One of the electrode strands was medial (toward the midline of the head) and the other was 4 mm. to the side of it.

Thomas's subjective responses to electrical stimuli delivered through the electrodes to points within the temporal lobe of his brain, are summarized in Figure 16. Repeated stimulations were made at each point, and each different response noted. Thomas had no way of knowing when or if we were stimulating the points on his electrode sheaths, and he had no notion of which points were being stimulated. Consequently, over a period of 10 weeks, we were able to stimulate points in a random pattern, and test the validity of each of his responses.

We used a number of different electrical currents to stimulate his brain. The most effective was a current with a pulse of 1 millisecond duration; it was a biphasic square wave delivered at a frequency of 50 cycles per second and was applied with

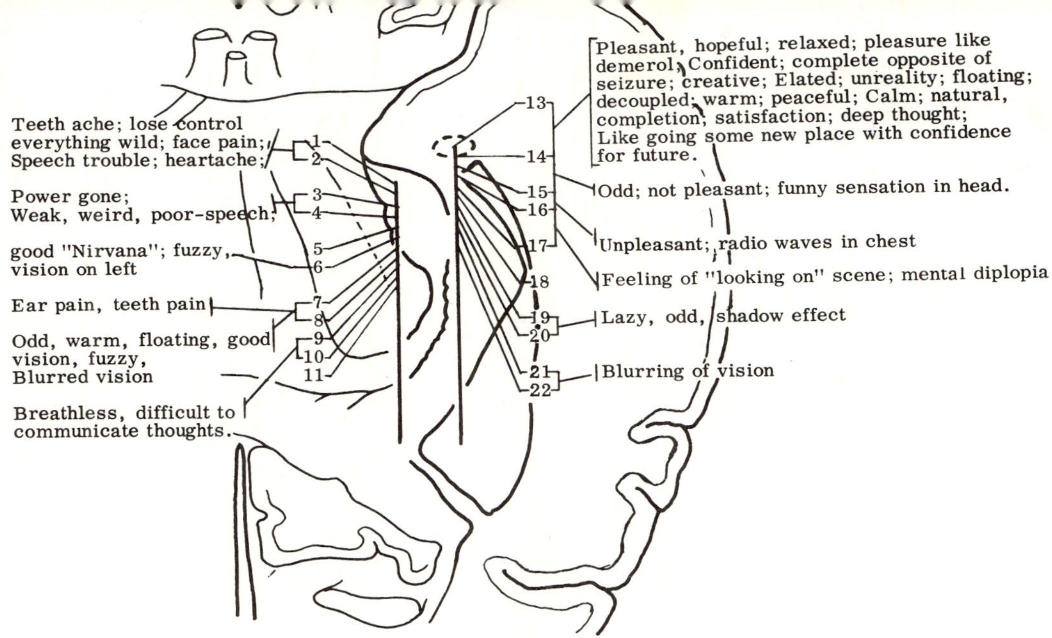

FIG. 16. Schematic drawing of electrode positions and responses to electrical stimuli in patient Thomas, showing left temporal lobe with two strands of inlying electrodes. Strand with electrodes 1-11 is toward midline of head; strand 13-22 is 4 mm. lateral. Electrodes 1 and 13 are anterior (toward the nose) and 11 and 22 are toward the back of the head. Patient's subjective verbal responses were produced by passing a weak stimulating current through the electrode points into adjacent brain tissue.

an intensity of 1 to 3 milliamperes. The individual trains of stimuli lasted 4 or 5 seconds. The central part of Figure 16 represents a schematic map of Thomas's verbal responses. There are two lines of dots which represent stimulation points side by side in the temporal lobe. The top of the two is anterior or just behind the eye; the bottom is posterior, toward the back of the head. The inner line of dots represents the responses elicited by passing a current through the electrodes in the more medial area of the amygdala (i.e., toward the midline of the head). This stimulation produced a complaint of pain, and a feeling of "I am losing control." We knew that both these reactions always marked the onset of one of Thomas's periods of violence, and since the electrodes we were then using had to be connected directly to large pieces of electronic equipment, we stimulated this area of the amygdala only twice for very short times to preclude any possibility of injury to him and ourselves—any sudden movement on his part might have broken or dislodged his brain electrodes.

Electrical stimulation through the electrodes 4 millimeters to the side produced an opposite response. It stopped Thomas's facial pain within 30 seconds, despite the fact that once his pains began they had always lasted from 2 to 4 hours. Within 60 to 90 seconds after the onset of stimulation, it also changed his mood from brooding preoccupation to relaxation. He reported this variously as a feeling of "hyperrelaxation," a "feeling like Demerol," "a feeling as though the room is getting larger and brighter," "I feel so relaxed," "I feel like I am floating on a cloud," and "I feel as though I am looking at the world through a television screen." This relaxed state did not disappear when the current was turned off, but instead dissipated slowly over a 4- to 18-hour period. Consequently, by stimulating the set of electrodes in his lateral amygdala every day, we were able to keep Thomas rage free for nearly 2 months.

However, it was obviously impractical to keep doing this for the rest of Thomas's life, and so we suggested to him that we make a destructive lesion in the medial portion of both his amygdalas—that is, in the area where stimulation elicited facial pain and rage. He agreed to this suggestion while he was relaxed from lateral stimulation of the amygdala. However, 12 hours later, when this effect had worn off, Thomas turned wild and unmanageable. The idea of anyone's making a destructive lesion in his brain enraged him. He absolutely refused any further therapy, and it took some weeks of patient explanation before he accepted the idea of bilateral lesions' being made in his medial amygdala. Four years have passed since the operation, during which time Thomas has not had a single episode of rage. He continues, however, to have an occasional epileptic seizure with periods of confusion and disordered thinking.

We saw and treated Julia S. nearly two years after Thomas had been discharged from the hospital. By then, we had perfected new techniques for identifying abnormal areas of electrical discharge in the brain. In addition, we were able to use the "stimoceiver"—the same telemetered device used to send signals and receive information from orbiting astronauts. Its application to clinical work was pioneered by Jose Delgado of Yale, who made the stimoceiver available to us.* Attaching the stimoceiver to implanted electrodes makes it possible to record or stimulate points deep within the brain touching the electrodes, from a distance of up to 100 feet without the use of connecting wires; and because the patient is unrestricted, this stimulation and recording can be carried out over a long period of time.

In Julia's case, the relationship between brain disease and violent behavior was very clear. Her history of brain disease went back to the time when, before the age of 2, she had a severe attack of encephalitis following mumps. When she was 10, she began to have epileptic seizures; occasionally these attacks were grand mal seizures. Most of the time, they consisted of brief lapses of consciousness, staring, lip smacking, and chewing. Often after such a seizure she would be overcome by panic and run off as fast as she could without caring about destination. Her behavior between seizures was marked by severe temper tantrums followed by extreme remorse. Four of these depressions ended in serious suicide attempts. The daughter of a professional man, she was an attractive, pleasant, cherubic blonde who looked much younger than her age of 21.

On twelve occasions, Julia had seriously assaulted other people without any apparent provocation. By far the most serious attack had occurred when she was 18. She was at a movie with her parents when she felt a wave of terror pass over her body. She told her father that she was going to have another one of her "racing spells" and agreed to wait for her parents in the ladies lounge. As she went to it, she automatically took a small knife out of her hand bag. She had gotten into the habit of carrying

* See *Appendix* on p. 109.

this knife for protection because her "racing spells" often took her into dangerous neighborhoods where she would come out of her fuguelike state to find herself helpless, alone, and confused. When she got to the lounge, she looked in the mirror and perceived the left side of her face and trunk (including the left arm) as shriveled, disfigured, and "evil." At the same time, she noticed a drawing sensation in her face and hands. Just then another girl entered the lounge and inadvertently bumped against Julia's left arm and hand. Julia, in a panic, struck quickly with her knife, penetrating the other girl's heart and then screamed loudly. Fortunately, help arrived in time to save the life of her victim.

The next serious attack occurred inside the mental hospital to which Julia had been sent. Julia's nurse was writing a report, and when Julia said "I feel another spell coming on, please help me," the nurse replied, "I'll be with you in just a minute." Julia dragged a pair of scissors out of the nurse's pocket and drove the point into the unfortunate woman's lungs. Luckily, the nurse recovered.

Julia's case clearly illustrates the point that violent behavior caused by brain dysfunction cannot be modified except by treating the dysfunction itself. She had had extensive medical care, and years' of psychotherapy. She had taken consecutively and in combination all the known antiseizure medications, as well as the entire range of drugs used to help emotionally disturbed patients. She had been treated in three of the major medical centers of North America with no sign of improvement. As a last resort, she had been given over sixty electroshock treatments, without any change in her seizures or in the pattern of her violence and rage.

The neurological examination made in our hospital showed Julia's ability to assimilate newly learned material was impaired, and, because of her shock treatments, she had a severe deficiency in both recent and remote memory. A brain wave examination disclosed a typical epileptic seizure pattern with spikes in both temporal regions, in addition to widespread abnormality over the rest of the brain. A special x-ray film of her brain disclosed some shrinkage of the tissue in the right temporal area.

Electrodes were placed stereotactically into both temporal lobes, and after she had recovered from the surgical procedure, we recorded epileptic electrical activity from both amygdalas.

Electrical stimulation of either amygdala produced symptoms characteristic of the beginning of her seizures. These symptoms were more easily elicited by stimulating her left amygdala, and therefore, a destructive lesion was made in the left temporal lobe in the region of the amygdala and all electrodes were withdrawn. However, her symptoms and seizures persisted and changed to include signs that indicated a small portion of her brain was firing abnormally, and that this area was related to the movement of her left arm (the one brushed against by the girl she stabbed). As the motor tract crosses over from one side of the brain to the opposite side of the body, this suggested that her persistent seizures and attack behavior were initiated in her right temporal lobe. Therefore, we again placed electrodes in her right amygdala.

By the time of this second operation, Dr. Delgado's "stimoceiver"* had become available to us, and we attached one to Julia's right temporal electrode. This device made it possible to record the electrical activity in her right amygdala and hippocampus from 100 feet away, while she moved around with others in her ward. We were thus able to observe the interactions between brain stimulations and environmental cues. We could also stimulate a selected target in her brain, from the same distance. Because there are no wires involved, we could try to reproduce her violent symptoms without fear that she might hurt herself by pulling out the electrodes, and we were also able to record the activity inside her brain continously for up to 24 to 36 hours.

The following records were made from this patient in a hospital room with the cooperation of Dr. Delgado. Both Julia and her parents knew that sometime during the day her brain was going to be recorded from and stimulated, but they had no idea when we were going to do it. Before we had done any stimulating, but while we were recording, the electrical activity recorded from the leads in Julia's amygdaloid nucleus showed a typical epileptic seizure pattern, as seen in Figure 17. The behavior that accompanied this change in Julia's brain waves involved her getting up and running over to the wall of her bedroom. Once there, she narrowed her eyes, bared her teeth, and clenched her fists—that is, she exhibited all the signs of being on the verge of making a physical attack.

The results of two episodes of electrical stimulation in her

* See *Appendix* on p. 109.

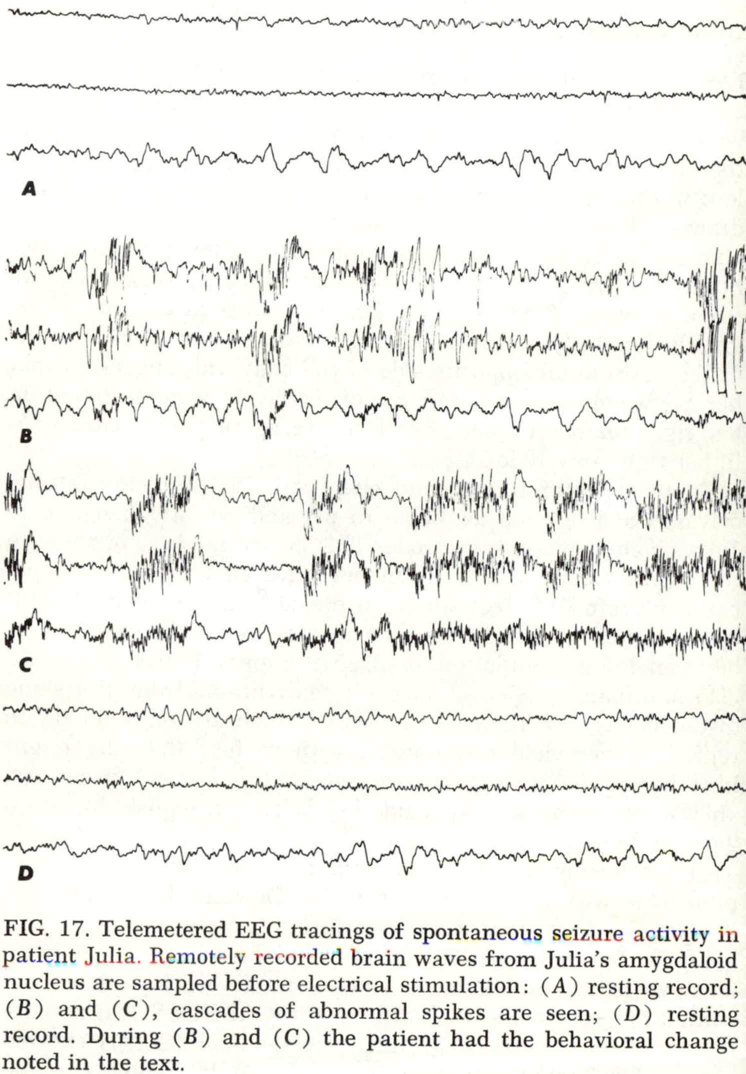

FIG. 17. Telemetered EEG tracings of spontaneous seizure activity in patient Julia. Remotely recorded brain waves from Julia's amygdaloid nucleus are sampled before electrical stimulation: (*A*) resting record; (*B*) and (*C*), cascades of abnormal spikes are seen; (*D*) resting record. During (*B*) and (*C*) the patient had the behavioral change noted in the text.

right amygdala can be seen in Figures 18 through 27. The stimulus was a five second train of 50 cycles per second biphasic square waves at one milliampere. Figure 18*A* shows the brain wave recordings in the resting state. There are three channels of recordings: the top represents the recordings from the electrode in the anterior amygdala, the second from the

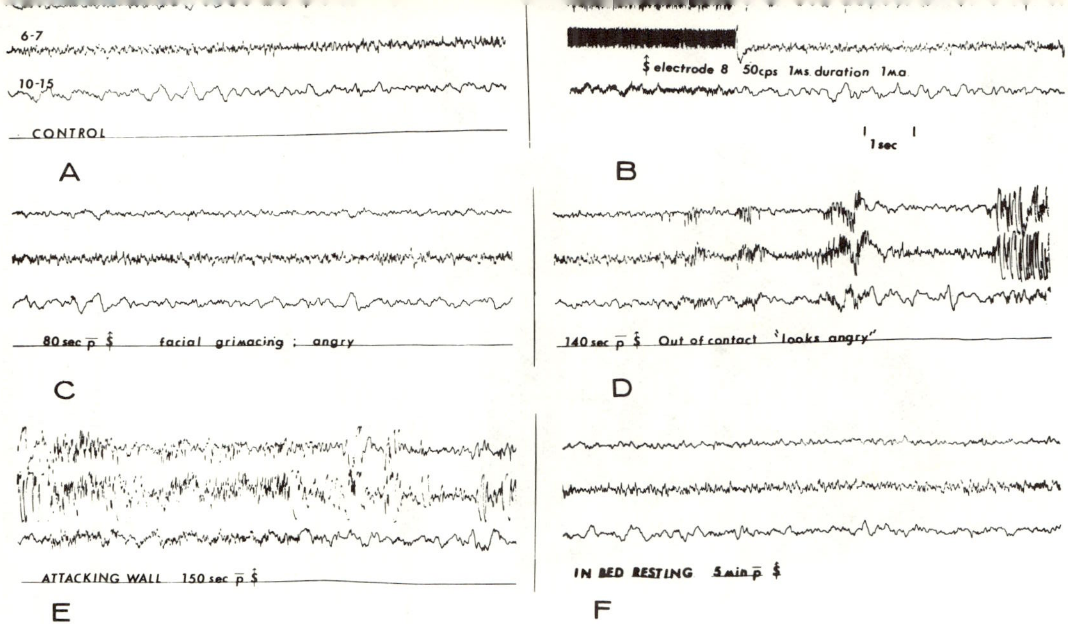

FIG. 18. Telemetered EEG tracings taken in Julia during episode in which she attacked the wall after stimulation. Remotely recorded brain waves from Julia's amygdala are seen in stimulus sequence: (*A*) Control recording (before stimulation); (*B*) amygdala is remotely stimulated with weak current; (*C*) electrical correlates of facial grimacing are not present; (*D*) cascades of spikes are followed by frank amygdaloid seizures which precede her attack behavior. (*E*) Her spring toward the wall occurs during amygdaloid seizure. (*F*) Five minutes after the attack behavior her brain wave record is similar to control recording.

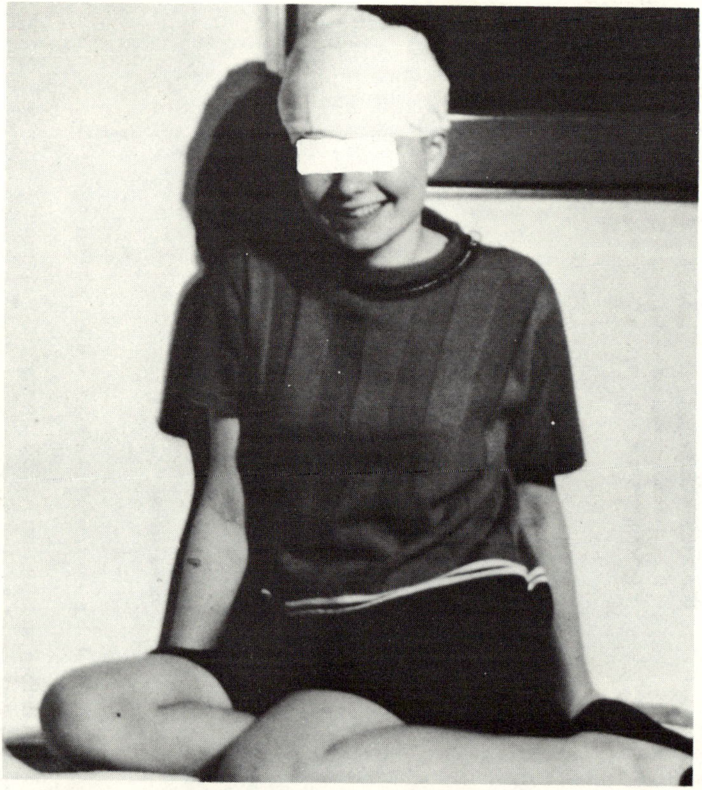

FIG. 19. Patient Julia in a pleasant mood. This photograph was taken from a motion picture sequence which was made simultaneously with the stimulation-recording sequence seen in Fig. 18. This shows her immediately before stimulation. (From LIFE Magazine, June 21, 1968.)

electrode in the posterior amygdala, and the third from an electrode in a part of the temporal lobe that is just behind the amygdala. In the first sequence, the electrical activity is near normal; then there is an interference pattern caused by the electrical stimulation (Fig. 18*B*); 130 seconds after the onset of stimulation, an occasional abnormal spike can be seen. At that point Julia was unresponsive to questioning. The next sequence, Figure 18*C* shows the electrical activity gradually becoming seizurelike; then a characteristic electrical epileptic seizure of the amygdala occurs. Immediately afterward, Julia exhibited rage behavior. The last tracing was taken 5 minutes

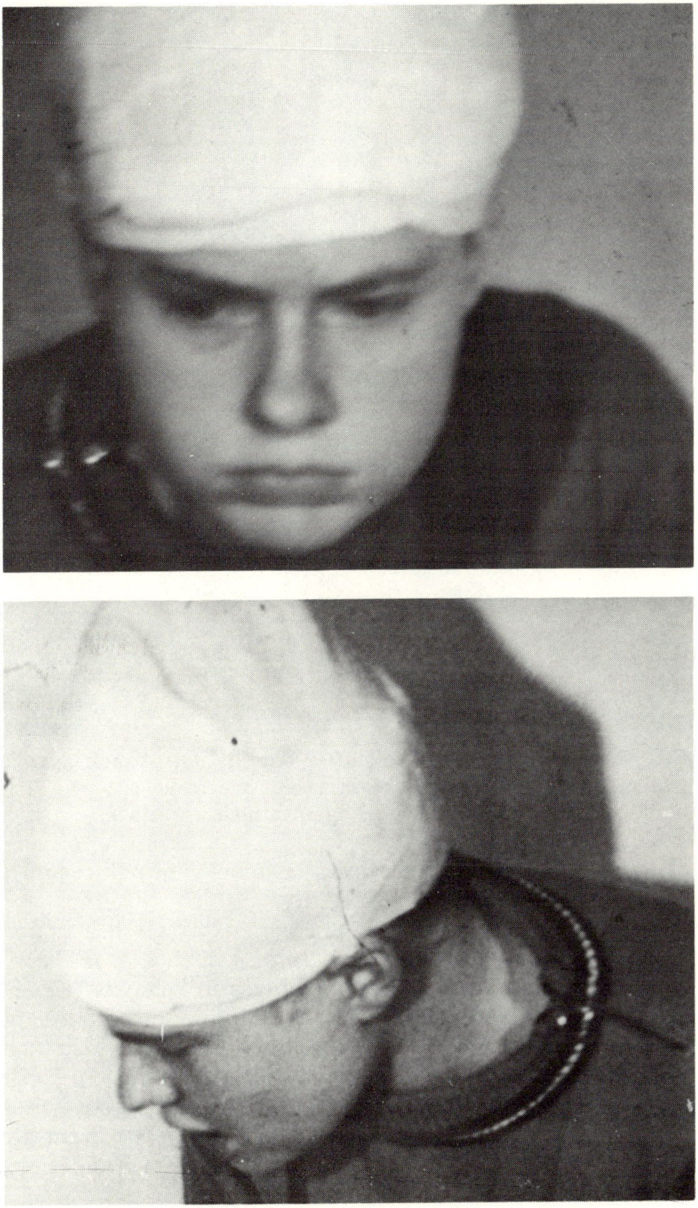

B

FIG. 20. *A*. Julia in an angry mood at onset of rage attack after stimulation. This shows the change in facial expression immediately following stimulation. *B*. Facial grimacing in this picture was followed by lip retraction and other signs of primate "threat display." (From LIFE Magazine June 21, 1968.)

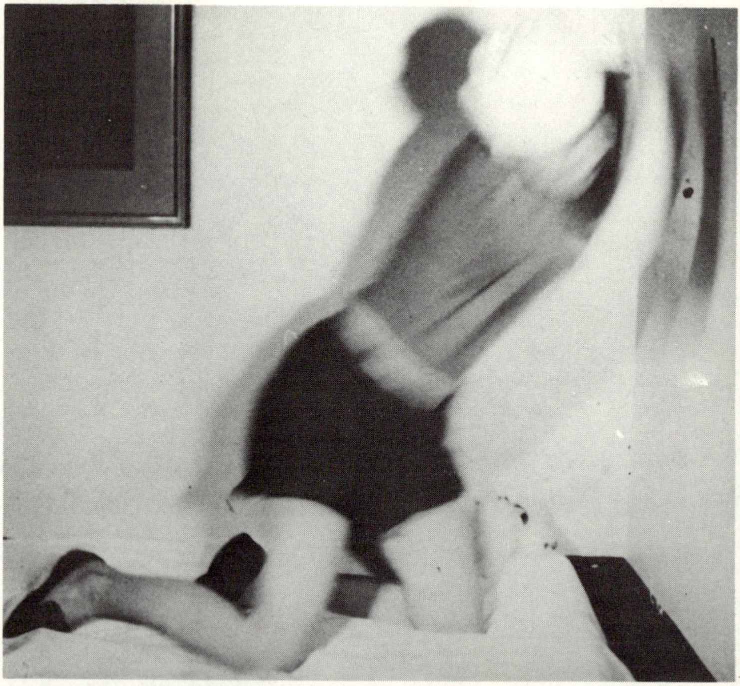

FIG. 21. Julia attacking wall after stimulation. Attack against the wall was both sudden and unexpected. We could see why it would be difficult to defend one's self against such an attack.

after stimulation and discloses a more normal record with some persistent postseizure activity.

A movie was made of Julia's actions while her brain was being stimulated, and the picture sequence has been abstracted to show the significant changes in behavior. Her initial behavior was placid (Fig. 19). After stimulation, she was out of contact, then she made a series of angry grimaces which included lip retraction and baring of the teeth, the ancient "primate threat display" (Figs. 20*A* and *B*). Her spring toward the wall was sudden and quite unexpected (Fig. 21). We were able to understand how victims of her attacks had not had the time to defend themselves!

The second stimulation sequence began while Julia was playing a guitar. Figures 22 and 23 show the brain wave recordings from the amygdala. The first recording, taken while the patient was singing and playing, was slightly abnormal (Fig. 22). The

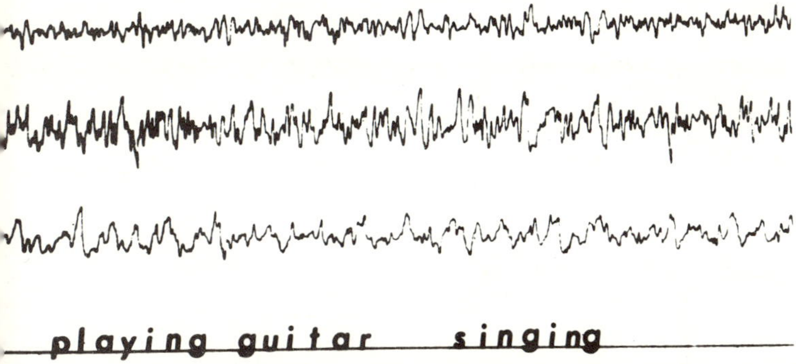

FIG. 22. Telemetered EEG tracings taken as Julia played her guitar and sang. Remote brain wave recordings were taken before another stimulation sequence.

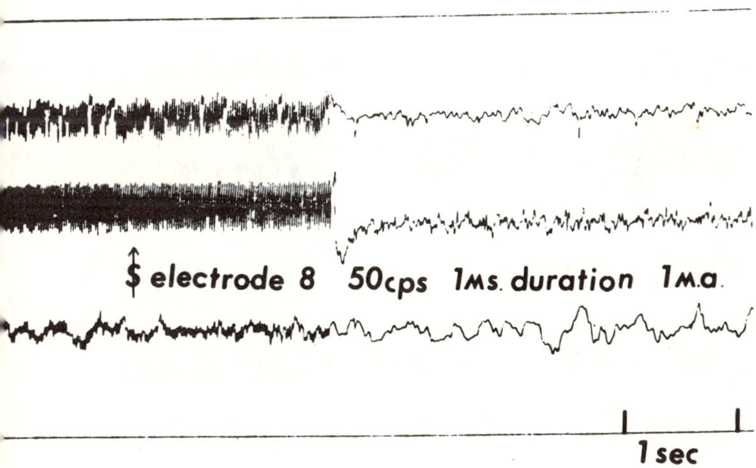

FIG. 23. Telemetered EEG tracings taken during and immediately after stimulation of the amygdala in patient Julia. Stimulation was carried out with immediate cessation of guitar playing and singing.

second recording shows the electrical artifact produced by the amygdala stimulation (Fig. 23). After 5 seconds of stimulation, Julia stopped singing and stared blankly ahead. During the next sequence she slipped out of communication and was unable to answer the questions posed by the psychiatrist who was examining her. A cascade of abnormal spikelike epileptic brain

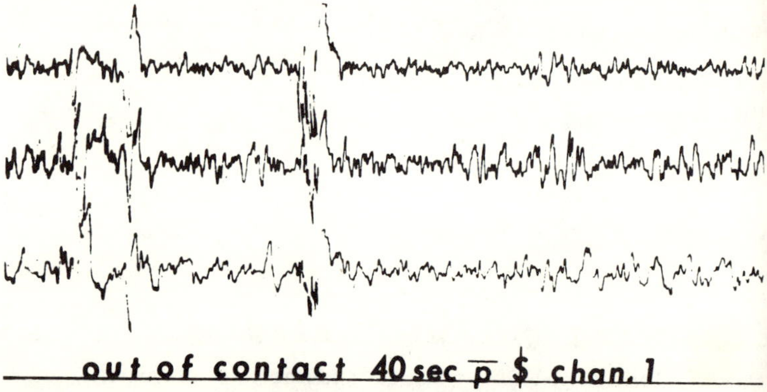

FIG. 24. Telemetered EEG tracings taken 40 seconds after amygdala stimulation shown in Fig. 23. Intermittent "abnormal spikes" in brain wave record; patient would not answer questions.

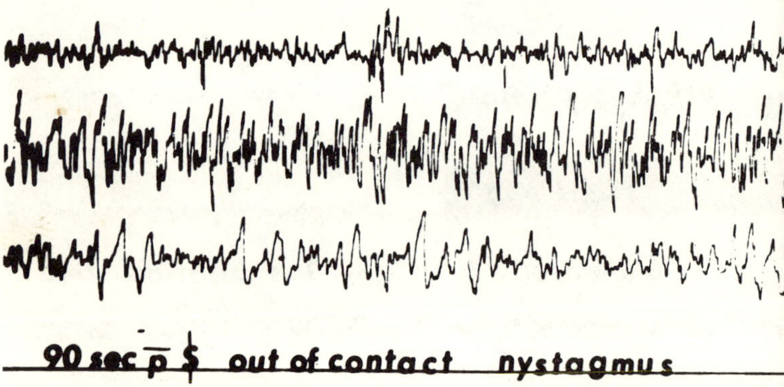

FIG. 25. Telemetered EEG tracings taken 90 seconds after stimulation shown in Fig. 23. Seizurelike brain wave activity is seen in second brain wave channel.

waves from her amygdala was then recorded (Fig. 24). The posterior amygdala exhibited a constant abnormal electrical discharge characteristic of seizure (Fig. 25). This was followed by a sudden and powerful swing of her guitar. She narrowly missed the head of the psychiatrist, and instead the guitar smashed against the wall (see Fig. 26). Her resting record shown in Figure 27, was taken later and showed only post-seizure slow wave activity.

A short time after these sequences were recorded, we made a

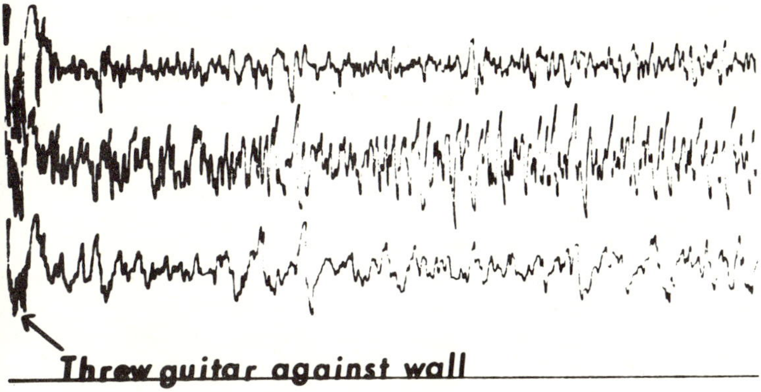

FIG. 26. Telemetered EEG tracings taken as Julia violently smashes her guitar against wall, narrowly missing the head of the examining psychiatrist. Seizurelike brain wave activity continues in her posterior amygdala.

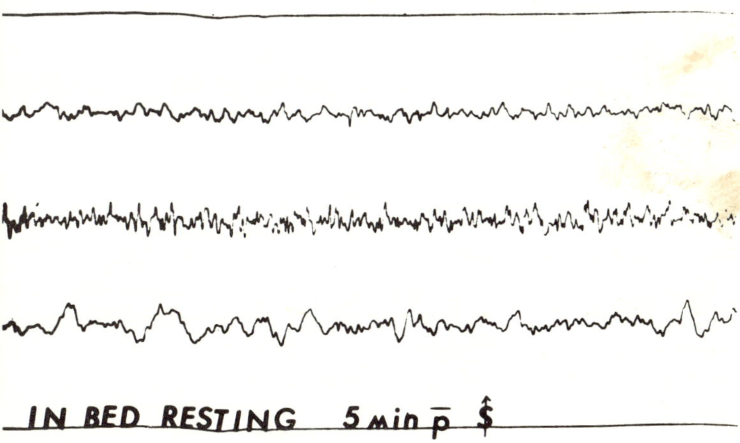

FIG. 27. Telemetered EEG tracings taken 5 minutes after stimulation shown in Fig. 23. Brain wave recordings are similar to prestimulation record. Third lead shows slower electrical waves, which may be postseizure in character.

destructive lesion in Julia's right amygdala. It is still too early to assess the results of the procedure, but she had only two mild rage episodes in the first postoperative year and none in the second. Since she had generalized brain disease and multiple areas of epileptic activity, it is not surprising that epileptic seizures have not been eliminated, or that her psychotic episodes have continued at the preoperative level.

The point we wish to make in this description of Julia's case is twofold. First: electrical stimulation of the amygdala initiated rage and violence; second: this behavior was preceded by the development of local electrical epileptic seizures. We are not maintaining that the amygdala—nor, indeed, the limbic system—is the only part of the brain involved in violent behavior. Our strands of electrodes are able to give us only a limited view of activity within the central nervous system, and other (perhaps many) areas of the brain must have been involved to produce such well-organized behavioral patterns. However, there can be no doubt that the electrical stimulation of and the abnormal seizure activity from the amygdala preceded and was directly related to Julia's violence. To our knowledge, this is the first time that rage behavior was artificially produced by electrical stimulation in an abnormal brain and used to diagnose the proper placement for a therapeutic lesion.

In summary, then, trigger areas exist in the human brain that can, *in susceptible individuals,* initiate violence if stimulated with a weak electric current. We also have evidence that the stimulation of neighboring points can inhibit violence—even when it has been initiated by stimulation. While this evidence is novel in relation to the human brain, it is not unexpected. The investigations with cats and monkeys described in Chapter 3 have evoked the same kinds of responses. We suspect—but cannot *prove* because of technical limitations—that the brain triggers and brakes for human violence are more varied, sophisticated, and subtle than similar mechanisms in lower animal forms. The idea, however, that strong basic brain mechanisms to suppress violence in the human are not present, or at best are "weak learned responses," is simply not substantiated by our investigations. Learning obviously modifies human behavior, but the basic mechanisms for the suppression of violence are present in every human being who has a normal brain.

REFERENCES

Bickford, R. G., Dodge, H. W., Jr., and Uhlein, A. Electrographic and Behavioral Effects Related to Depth Stimulation in Human Patients." In: *Electrical Studies on the Unanesthetized Brain.* (E. R. Ramey and D. S. O'Doherty, eds.). New York, Hoeber, 1960.

Chapman, W. P., Schroeder, H. R., Geyer, G., Brazier, M. A. B., Fager, C., Poppen, J. L., Solomon, H. C., and Yakovlev, P. I. Physiological evidence concerning importance of the amygdaloid region in the integration of circulatory function and emotion in man. *Science 120:* 949–950, 1954.

Delgado, J. M. R. Control of behavior by electronic stimulation of the brain. *Naval Res. Rev.* May: 1–7, 1959.

Delgado, J. M. R. Electronic command of movement and behavior. *Trans. NY Acad. Sci. (Ser. II) 21:*689–699, 1959.

Delgado, J. M. R. Modification of social behavior induced by remote-controlled electrical stimulation of the brain. *XXI Int. Congr. Physiol. Sci.* (Abst.), p. 75, 1959.

Delgado, J. M. R. Prolonged stimulation of brain in awake monkeys. *J. Neurophysiol.* 22:458–475, 1959.

Delgado, J. M. R. Chronic radiostimulation of the brain in monkey colonies. *Proc. Int. Union Physiol. Sci. 4:*365–371, 1965.

Delgado, J. M. R. Evoking and inhibiting aggressive behavior by radio stimulation in monkey colonies. *Amer. Zool. 5:*642, 1965.

Delgado, J. M. R. Aggressive behavior evoked by radio stimulation in monkey colonies. *Amer. Zool. 6:*669–681, 1966.

Delgado, J. M. R. "Aggression and Defense Under Cerebral Radio Control." In: *Aggression and Defense: Neural Mechanisms and Social Patterns.* UCLA Forum in Medical Science No. 7, Vol. V (C. D. Clemente and D. B. Lindsley, eds.). Berkeley: Univ. California Press, pp. 171–193, 1967.

Delgado, J. M. R., Mark, V. H., Sweet, W. H., Ervin, F. R., Gerhardt, W., Bach-y-Rita, G., and Hagiwara, R. Intracerebral radio stimulation and recording in completely free patients. *J.Nerv. Ment. Dis. 147:* 329–340, 1968.

Ervin, F. R., Mark, V. H., and Stevens, J. R. Behavioral and affective responses to brain stimulation in man. *Amer. Psychopath. Ass. Trans.* 1968.

Ervin, F. R., Mark, V. H., and Sweet, W. H. Focal cerebral disease, temporal lobe epilepsy and violent behavior. *Trans. Amer. Neurolog. Ass. 94:*253–256, 1969.

Heath, R. G. Electrical self-stimulation of the brain in man. *Amer. J. Psychiat. 120:*571–577, 1963.

Heath, R. G. (ed.) *The Role of Pleasure in Behavior.* New York, Hoeber, 1964.

Heath, R. G., and Guerrero-Figueroa, R. Psychotic behavior with evoked septeal dysrrthmia: Effects of intracerebral acetycholine and gamma-amnobutyric acid. *Amer. J. Psychiat. 121:*1080, 1965.

Mark, V. H., Ervin, F. R., Sweet, W. H., and Delgado, J. M. R. Remote telemeter stimulation and recording from implanted temporal lobe electrodes. *Confin. Neurol. 31*:86–93, 1969.

Mark, V. H., Barry, H., McLardy, T., and Ervin, F. R. The destruction of both anterior thalamic nuclei in a patient with intractable agitated depression. *J. Nerv. Ment. Dis. 150*:266–272, 1970.

Stevens, J. R., Mark, V. H., Ervin, F. R., Pacheco, P., and Suematsu, K. Long latency, long lasting psychological changes induced by deep temporal stimulation in man. *Archt. Neurol. 21*:157–169, 1969.

Appendix

The tools designed by Dr. Jose Delgado for remote stimulation and recording in patients with inlying depth electrodes make it possible both to stimulate and to record deep focal areas of the brain without direct wire connections between the tiny instrument attached to the electrode in the patient's head and the stationary electronic stimulating and recording device. The instrument consists of two parts: the first is the stimulator, which in turn consists of two parts: (a) radiofrequency transmitter, which is not attached to the patient and which has the circuitry for controlling the repetition rate, the duration, and the intensity of the stimulating pulse, and (b) the receiver, which is attached to the electrode on the patient's head, and measures 3.7 × 3 × 1.4 cm. and weighs 20 gm. The receiver contains solid-state circuitry which enables it to detect the radiofrequency signal and demodulate it into the ordinary stimulating current. A constant circuit transistor in the output circuit makes the pulse intensity independent of biological impedance changes over a wide range. Three channels of stimulation are available, and the operating range is up to 100 feet.

The second part of the instrument capsule is used for recording the brain activity generated around the depth electrodes. It consists of a miniature FM amplifier-FM transmitter combination, and the telemetering receiver. The transmitting circuitry carried by the patient consists of this amplifier with a gain of 100 and input impedance of 2 megaohms; it has a frequency response from 2 to 200 cycles per second and a voltage control oscillator for each of 3 recording channels. The miniaturized radiofrequency transmitter operates at 216 megacycles and its range is 50 to 200 feet, depending on the environment. The size of this 3 channel unit including the battery is 4.5 × 4.5 × 1.5 cm and it weighs 50 gm. It sends a radiofrequency signal to a unit which demodulates this into telemetered analog information, which can be delivered into the input of a regular brain wave machine amplifier. In our case, these analog signals were fed to the inputs of a brain wave machine and a magnetic tape recorder. The entire instrument, weighing 70 gm, can be taped into the patient's head bandage.

Chapter 8

Hidden Brain Disease

Appearances are deceptive.

Aesop
The Wolf in Sheep's Clothing

All the persons we have described thus far were known to have brain disease, which, as we have shown, proved to be related to their violent behavior. But what of those individuals who are uncontrollably violent but do *not* have epileptic seizures or other obvious signs of brain disease? They are just as apt to be dangerous to other drivers as Thomas R. and they are as quick to defend themselves against what they perceive as a threat as Julia or Clara. Is it possible that they, too, are suffering from an abnormality of the limbic system? And is there any way we can identify them as being potentially violent?

One girl for whom these questions were not academic was Jennie—a double murderess at the age of 14. She came from a broken home, and had been brought up by an aunt and uncle. She had three younger stepsisters. Till she was 13, Jennie was a model child—dependable and responsible with the younger children.

Jennie's troubles* began on New Year's Eve of the year that

* We are grateful to Dr. William H. Sweet for his permission to describe his patient Jennie W. in this chapter.

she was 13. Her aunt told her to turn down the volume on her record player, to which Jennie reacted by going beserk. She smashed the furniture in her room, broke windows, and created such a disturbance that the police had to be called. Shortly after this, while she was babysitting with her stepsisters, she was very disturbed by one youngster's constant crying, so she put a plastic bag over the child's head and suffocated her. Jennie was frightened by what she'd done and ran to a girl friend's house, where the police found her. Because her action was so senseless, and because she was so young, she was sent to a mental institution for observation. While she was being questioned by a psychiatrist there, she confessed that she had also killed another younger stepsister who was thought to have died of pneumonia.

The physicians at the state hospital did a thorough medical and psychiatric examination without finding any abnormality; the opinion of the psychiatric staff at the state hospital was that Jennie in *no way differed* from hundreds of other prisoners accused of a serious crime. Nonetheless they decided to have a neurologist review her case—partly because she was so young, partly because of a brother with known epilepsy, and also because she had had a good behavior record before she committed the two murders. The neurologist felt intuitively, rather than on the basis of any definite evidence, that Jennie had temporal lobe disease and should be studied further. She was, therefore, referred into the Massachusetts General Hospital for further evaluation.

In the hospital, the results of neurological and psychiatric examinations were inconclusive, and her brain-wave examinations disclosed no definite abnormality. Psychological tests indicated that Jennie was a "dull-normal" girl. The psychologist's diagnosis was that she had a character disorder.

Special x-ray films of the brain showed that the fluid-filled space within the left temporal lobe (temporal horns) was somewhat deformed (Fig. 28). Even though this configuration often indicates a tumor, we did not want to remove her temporal lobe on this evidence alone and decided to record directly from the surface of the temporal lobe by inserting tiny electrodes through the skull and placing them on the surface of the brain. At the same time, stereotactic electrodes were implanted on each side of her brain through the temporal lobe and into the nucleus amygdala. The special x-ray techniques used to guide the elec-

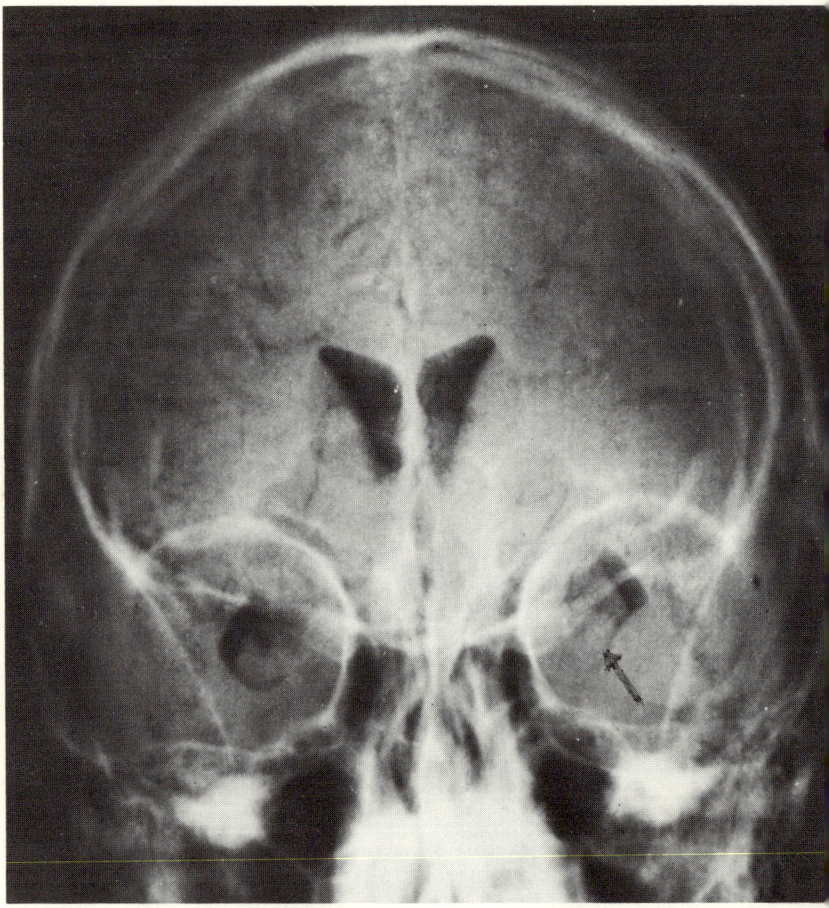

FIG. 28. X-ray film with air in ventricles of patient Jennie suggests abnormality of left temporal horn. Outline of temporal (ventricular) horn on left seems to be abnormal. Spaces inside brain (ventricles) are filled with air. Later x-ray, taken during stereotactic surgery, showed ventricle and horn to be normal.

trodes to their proper target within the temporal lobe did not, however, reveal the brain abnormalities seen on the previous films.

At this point, then, Jennie had electrodes on the surface of her temporal lobe and within the temporal lobe itself. But the results of the neurological examination, the brain wave examina-

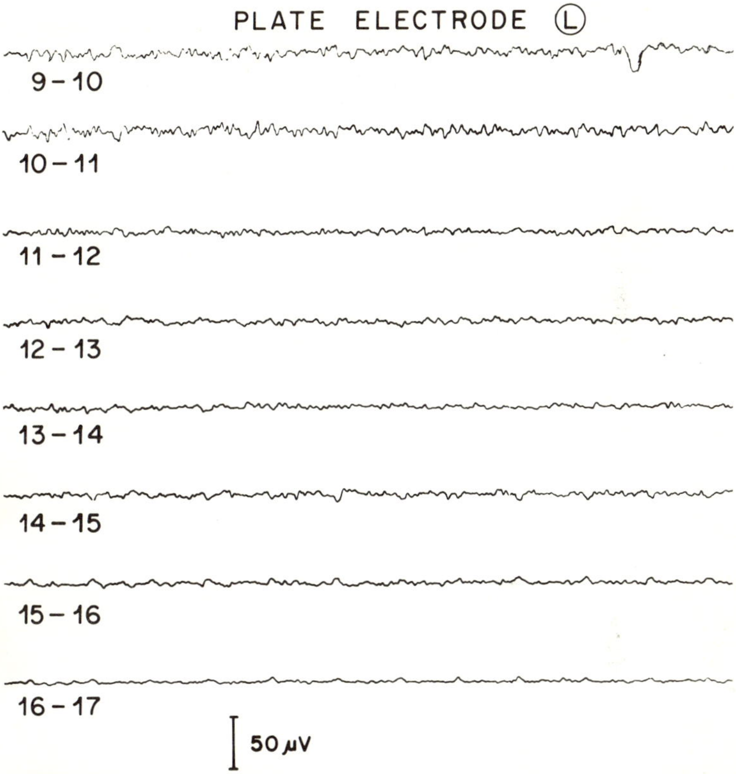

FIG. 29. Telemetered EEG tracings taken directly from surface of brain of patient Jennie. Brain wave recording from surface of temporal lobe are normal.

tion, the brain scan, and the final x-ray films of her brain were all normal. The primary evidence that supported the idea she might have brain disease was that she had murdered two children.

When Jennie had recovered from surgery, a careful examination was made of the brain wave recordings from the implanted electrodes. The brain waves recorded from the surface of the temporal lobe itself are reproduced in Figure 29. They are quite normal. The recordings from the amygdala are also normal (Figs. 30 and 31). But the recordings from the electrode directly in the hippocampus were strikingly abnormal (Figs. 32 and 33). These records show localized epileptic discharges.

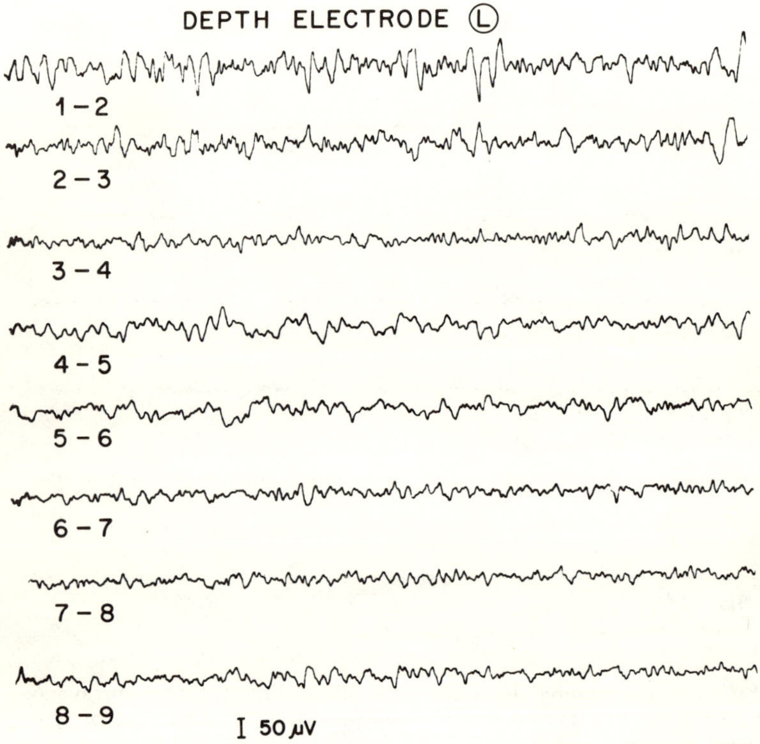

FIG. 30. Telemetered EEG tracings from left amygdala of patient Jennie. Brain wave recordings from left amygdala appear normal.

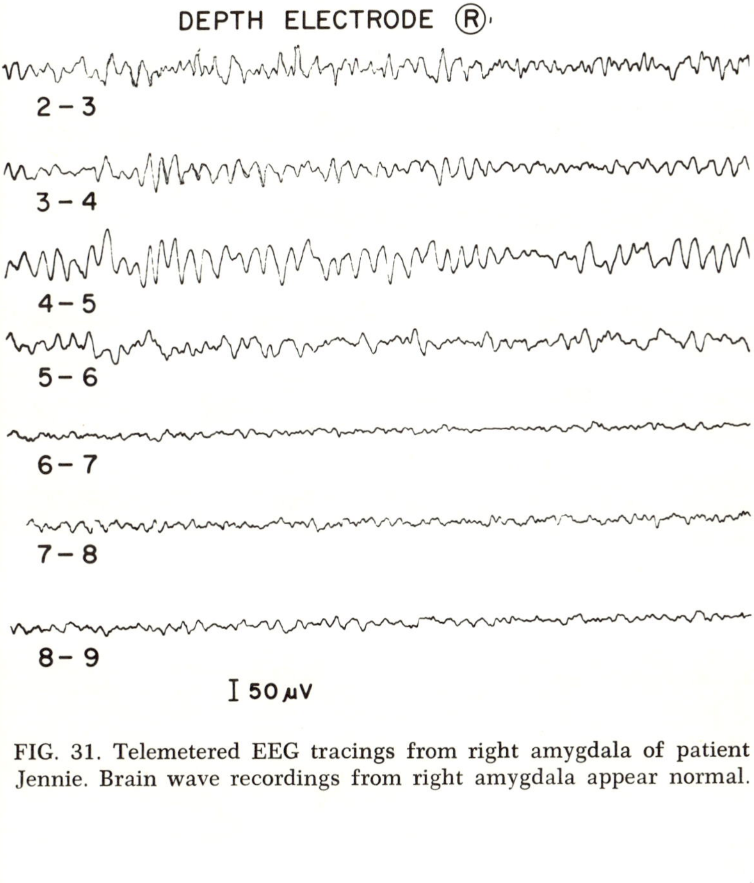

FIG. 31. Telemetered EEG tracings from right amygdala of patient Jennie. Brain wave recordings from right amygdala appear normal.

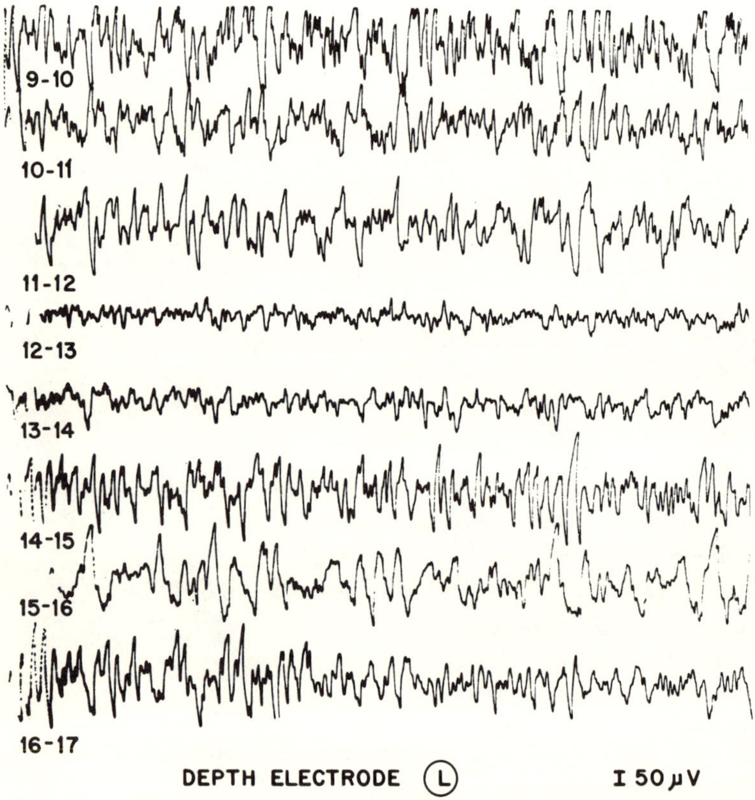

FIG 32. Telemetered EEG tracings from left hippocampus of patient Jennie. Brain wave recordings from deep areas of temporal lobe behind amygdala are quite abnormal and are unlike hippocampal spindles. There is, in fact, a seizurelike pattern present.

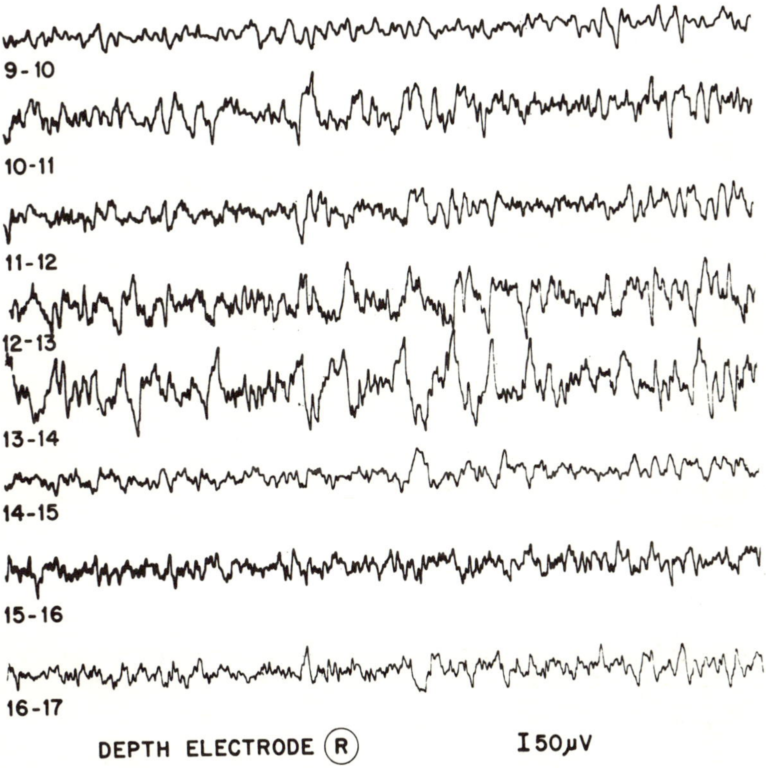

FIG. 33. Telemetered EEG tracings from right hippocampus of patient Jennie. Right posterior leads also show marked abnormalities, especially in leads 11-12 and 12-13.

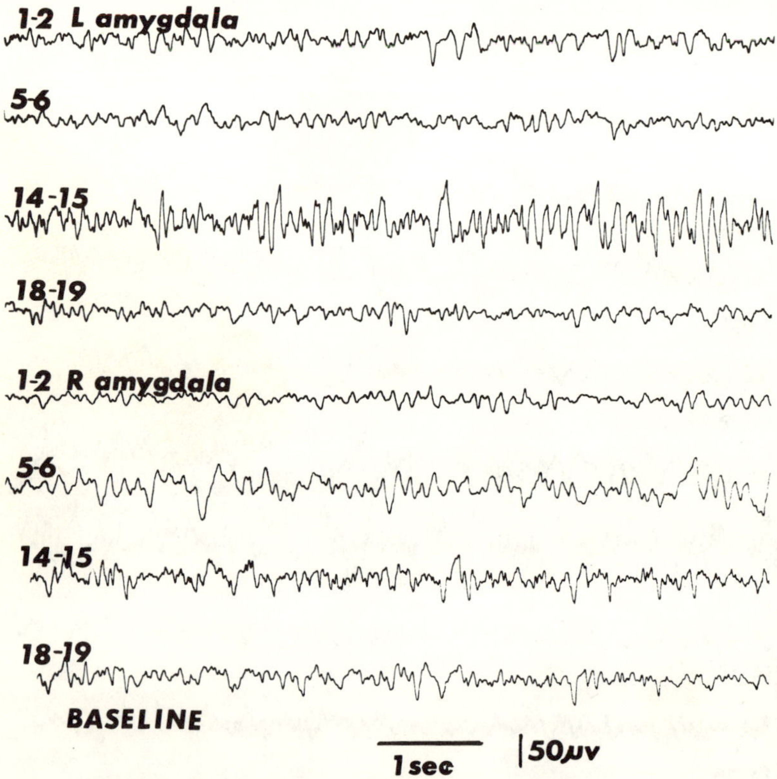

FIG. 34. Telemetered EEG tracings from patient Jennie before she hears recording of baby crying. Brain wave recording from both right and left temporal lobes was taken before turning on tape recording.

We knew that a baby's cry was able to provoke an extreme behavioral change in Jennie. In fact, when she was in the state hospital, she could not be left alone with a young child because if it cried Jennie would become vicious. We decided, therefore, to play a tape of a baby's cry while we were recording electrical activity from the depths of both of her temporal lobes. This taped stimulus elicited a marked behavioral response of discomfort and anxiety; it also provoked a burst of electrical seizure activity from her temporal lobe (Figs. 35–37). Furthermore, electrical stimulation in this same region produced a typical temporal lobe seizure with staring and with what Jennie described as a "waving, floating, feeling." The brain wave record-

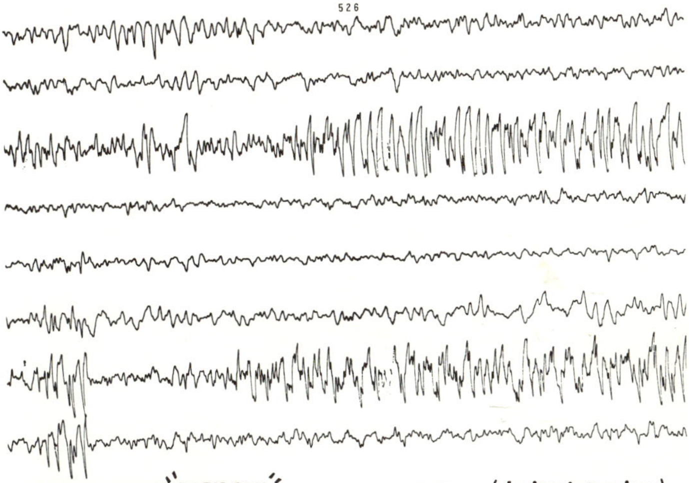

FIG. 35. Telemetered EEG tracings from patient Jennie 40 seconds after onset of a recording of baby crying. Brain wave abnormality which occurred after patient heard the taped cry was more pronounced in posterior leads.

ings from her medial temporal lobe, taken immediately after the stimulation disclosed findings typical of seizure activity. Jennie reported that her floating feelings recurred several times after the stimulation had stopped, and later on told us she had experienced them before but never mentioned them because she "thought that everyone had them."

Jennie was given anticonvulsant medication while she was in our care; after her electrodes were removed, she was sent to a state institution, where unfortunately, we had no authority to keep on with what we believed was necessary medical treatment.

Jennie's case is significant for two reasons. First, it shows that violent, irrational behavior may be the only overt symptom of brain disease, especially when the abnormalities are deep within the brain and do not register on brain wave recordings from the scalp, or even from the outer surface of the brain itself. Secondly, it proves that we need, but do not yet have, some accurate method of identifying people with deep brain disease, preferably before they commit any violent act, but certainly, at least, before they commit more than one. It is obvious that we must develop some routine way to test for limbic brain function

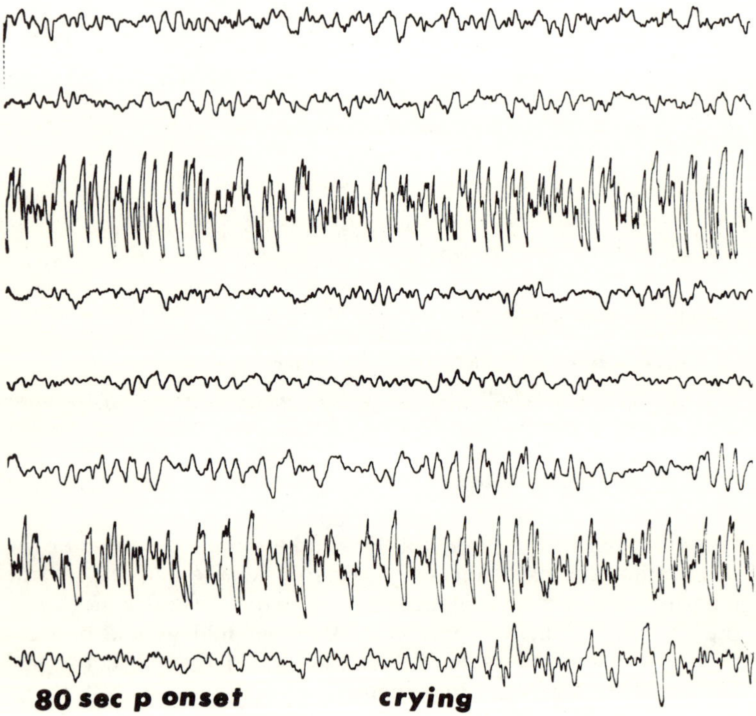

FIG. 36. Telemetered EEG tracings from patient Jennie 80 seconds after onset of recording of baby crying. Brain wave abnormality has persisted for more than 80 seconds and is still most evident in posterior leads. Patient is quite angry.

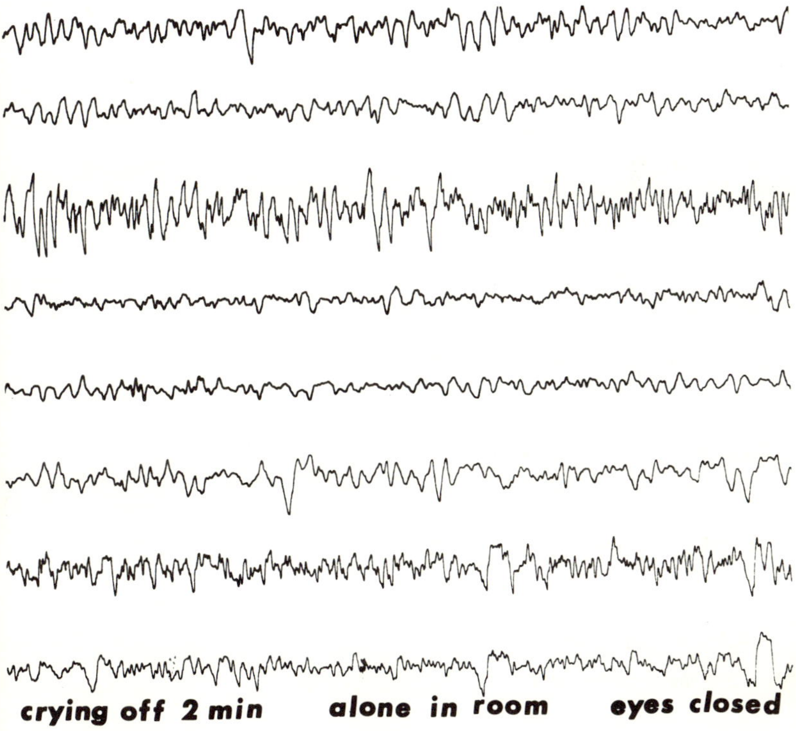

FIG. 37. Telemetered EEG tracings from patient Jennie 2 minutes after recording of baby crying is turned off. Brain wave recording is becoming more normal after 2 minutes, but posterior leads still contain abnormal recordings.

and malfunction. Without such a test, we cannot hope to detect, predict, or prevent individual violence related to limbic brain disease.

REFERENCES

Ervin, F. R., Mark, V. H., and Sweet, W. H. Focal cerebral disease, temporal lobe epilepsy and violent behavior. *Trans. Amer. Neurolog. Ass.* *94*:253–256, 1969.

Sweet, W. H., Ervin, F. R., and Mark, V. H. The Relationship of Violent Behavior to Focal Cerebral Disease. In: *Aggressive Behavior* (S. Garattini and E. B. Sigg, eds.). Amsterdam, Excerpta Medica Foundation, pp. 336–352, 1969.

Chapter 9

The Dyscontrol Syndrome

Oh this poor brain. Ten thousand shapes of fury are whirling there, and reason is no more.

Henry Fielding

Since we do not at present have any way to test directly for the presence of limbic brain disease, we must rely on two indirect methods of diagnosis. The first is to see if the violent person has any signs and symptoms of recognizable brain disease—especially any signs of abnormality in a part of the brain which is close to the limbic brain. We know, for example, that difficulty in reading and speaking may be related to an abnormality in the temporal lobe; also, a disturbance in remote or recent memory may be related to an abnormality in the medial temporal lobe. In addition, a partial loss of sight may be caused by a dysfunction of the portions of the visual pathways that traverse the temporal lobe. Other evidence of limbic brain disease may include symptoms of temporal lobe epilepsy as well as hallucinations, feelings of panic, or severe unexplained depression.

The second indirect way to identify violent persons with limbic brain disease is to compare their behavior with that of people known to have this sort of disease. At the Massachusetts

General Hospital, we first reviewed the histories of our patients known to have limbic brain disease and temporal lobe epilepsy, paying close attention to those with implanted electrodes, and especially seeking signs of poor impulse control (which most of these people might have in common). We then checked the symptoms we found such patients did share against the histories of 108 self-referred patients at the Massachusetts General Hospital and 24 patients at the Boston City Hospital, all of whom had a principal complaint of poor impulse control with periods of destructive behavior. We also checked our list against the histories of more than 400 violent prisoners in a large penitentiary.

We found that these violent people usually had four characteristic symptoms, (which were not, however, always present at the same time): (1) a history of physical assault, especially wife and child beating; (2) the symptom of pathological intoxication—that is, drinking even a small amount of alcohol triggers acts of senseless brutality;* (3) a history of impusive sexual behavior, at times including sexual assaults; and (4) a history (in those who drove cars) of many traffic violations and serious automobile accidents. We shall refer to this set of symptoms together as "the dyscontrol syndrome."

Our findings are not unique, for other researchers have also observed them in the histories of individuals suffering from poor impulse control. Karl Menninger and his co-workers, for instance, in describing the disorders of impulse control from a psychodynamic point of view, defined one order of dyscontrol as "ego rupture" manifested by two general syndromes: (1) the chronic, repetitious occurrence of relatively milder (although serious) aggression, and (2) sudden, explosive outbursts of very serious aggression. Dr. Russell Monroe in his recent book describes in detail the various facets of the dyscontrol syndrome.

Our observation that any single act of violence is not isolated, atypical behavior, but one in a series of violent incidents is supported by Wolfgang's study of 588 homicides committed in Philadelphia. He found that homicide is generally preceded by a number of other violent acts. In 550 of the homicides, the

* There is some evidence that in pathological intoxication the act of drinking, rather than the alcohol itself, is the stimulus for brutality. Individuals who become violent after taking even a small amount of liquor by mouth may be injected intravenously with enough alcohol to produce clinical drunkenness without any sign of violent behavior.

assailants were known; 64 per cent of these murderers had a previous arrest record, and of these 66 per cent had a record of crimes against persons, with 75 per cent having committed aggravated assault. In England, D. J. West discovered that even murder may not be the last in the series of violent acts, for one-third of the prisoners apprehended for murder later committed suicide.

As for consistent recurrence of traffic violence, a recent analysis of traffic accidents and violations (summarized in the *Journal of the American Medical Association*) showed that drivers with a history of epilepsy or of fainting spells are more apt to violate traffic rules or have automobile accidents than other drivers.* Both Willett, in *Criminal on the Road*, and Storr, in *Human Aggression*, confirm our findings that violence, sex crimes, and dangerous driving often occur together. In Great Britain there is a chance of nearly one in three that a motorist guility of a serious driving offense will already be known to the police as a person suspected of some crime, or he will have a record of a previous conviction for a nonmotoring offense.

The easiest and clearest way to illustrate the characteristics of the dyscontrol syndrome is by citing a few pertinent histories. Before doing so, we must repeat that although the three cases we describe here have signs of temporal lobe abnormality, we do not mean to imply either that all people with brain disease are violent, nor that all those people who are violent have brain disease. We do believe, however, that brain dysfunction affecting the limbic system is more apt to be related to the dyscontrol syndrome than disease in other areas of the brain. Further, it is significant that in two of these three cases we were able to alleviate the symptoms of dyscontrol with anticonvulsant medications.

A good example of the dyscontrol syndrome was Tony D. who suffered from pathological intoxication. He had a history of recurrent brutality, wife beating, and sexual assault, and had been involved in near-fatal car crashes. He was a husky 25-year-old skilled machinist who had been sent to a hospital for the criminally insane after assaulting his mistress and fracturing a

* The occurrence of driver intoxication in a significant number of serious or fatal auto accidents is well documented. And, of course, an intoxicated brain is by definition a malfuntioning brain. *Furthermore, recent evidence indicates that limbic structures are sensitive to the effect of alcohol.*

number of her facial bones. He had also beaten his wife many times; once he had hit her with a lead pipe, another time he had tried to knife her. His wife also told us that he had tried to smother their infant son with a pillow. He became violent after drinking even a small amount of alcohol. To study alcohol's effect, we gave Tony one drink while recording his brain waves; he promptly grew so violent we had to stop the brain wave examination. Tony's drinking usually started with an auditory hallucination—like the voice of his dead father telling him to kill his brother—and culminated in physical violence, often directed against his wife and child.

Tony had suffered a serious head injury while driving a car. His neurological examination disclosed that although he had normal intelligence, he was quite unable to read and could write his name only with difficulty. It also revealed bilateral temporal lobe brain wave abnormalities. He was treated with Dilantin, an anticonvulsant medication, which produced a marked improvement in his behavior. We were not able to see if the improvement kept up because he refused to return for a follow-up examination and there was no way for us to compel him to continue with treatment.

The history of 38-year-old Theresa L. illustrates the sexual aspects of the dyscontrol syndrome. Even in an era of increasingly liberal social codes, her activities were unusual enough to attract attention. When we first saw her, she was in the psychiatric ward of the Boston City Hospital; and in this open ward setting, she was masturbating 18 to 20 times a day. She had a history of promiscuous sexual relations with lesbian prostitutes; she would also go to bed with two or more men at a time and exhaust them all with her demands. Her extreme promiscuity and her indiscriminate use of any thing or any body as a source of sexual gratification is reminiscent of the behavior of the monkeys with bilateral temporal lobectomies described in Chapter 3. Unlike these placid animals, however, Theresa was dangerous. She was abusive and assaultive to other patients on the ward and to the attendants. She had attempted to emasculate her husband with the edge of a broken bottle, and had cut the back of another man with a razor.

Prolonged psychiatric treatment was ineffective, and an astute psychiatric resident requested a brain wave examination which disclosed generalized brain abnormalities with a focus of abnormal brain waves in the right frontal temporal region. Theresa was given Dilantin. Her sexual activity immediately decreased, and this improvement continued as long as she took her daily dose of medication. Unfortunately, she refused to take it faithfully, and twice during periods when she went off it, she attempted suicide.

Traffic violence as an aspect of the dyscontrol syndrome is graphically illustrated in the history of 25-year-old Fred F. He had had encephalitis as an infant, and had also suffered a severe head injury while serving in the Navy. Following his discharge from the service, he began to have spells of temporal lobe epilepsy characterized by staring, lip smacking, stereotyped hand movements, and mumbling of incoherent, inappropriate words and phrases. Fred's history included assaults made on both men and women.

On one occasion when he was driving a large trailer truck, Fred blacked out in the middle of Los Angeles and did not come to until he was on the outskirts of Reno. He had a similar experience while riding a motorcycle. Although nothing untoward happened during either of these two episodes, another time he did kill someone in a head-on collision. He also had been given a number of traffic citations for lesser violations.

Fred was admitted to a Veteran's Administration Hospital, and had a complete neurological and psychiatric examination. Brain wave examinations disclosed focal epileptic abnormalities in both temporal regions and an x-ray examination of his brain disclosed right temporal lobe shrinkage. After an initial period of cooperation, he began to assault both nurses and doctors, and had to be transferred to a mental institution. A prolonged trial of various anticonvulsant and tranquilizing drugs had no effect on the number of seizures or on his tendency to make unprovoked assaults; he was therefore transferred to Massachusetts General Hospital for temporal lobe electrode implantation.

After these operations, brain wave recordings showed particularly prominent abnormalities in the right temporal lobe. Electrical stimulation of his right amygdala (through the implanted electrodes) produced remarkable changes in his mood and thought processes. These amygdala stimulations were repeated, and the number of seizures diminished to the point where we decided it was unnecessary to destroy any of his brain cells. Therefore, we took the electrodes out and started him on a program of rehabilitation therapy. He made good progress for about a year. Then he went through three months during which the number of his seizures increased and he began to drink. Changes in his medication, as well as in his surroundings, helped to reduce both the frequency of his seizures and the bouts of alcoholism. Fred has not had his driver's license renewed, however, we feel that it is not in his or the public's interest that he be allowed to get behind the wheel of a car!

Our study of the dyscontrol syndrome among the 154 patients and more than 400 prisoners presented some interesting contrasts and similarities.

Of the 108 patients examined at the Massachusetts General Hospital, only 83 were available for a detailed psychiatric, neurological, and laboratory examination. These 83 were not necessarily the sickest or most violent individuals, because extremely disorganized and violent patients were sent to psychiatric hospitals during their acute turmoil. A small number of the 108 had been arrested and were unable to complete their examination. Others in this group of restless, anxious, and impulsive people found it impossible to sustain the tedium of a series of thorough biomedical examinations in the out-patient department, and were lost to follow-up.

Of the 83 self-referred patients who were available for detailed examination, 10 consulted us about violent feelings directed at another specific individual—for example, wife, father, or brother. Although they may have committed physical assault on others also, it seemed likely that the best way to approach these people initially was to try and understand their relationships to the target individuals. The remaining 73, although they most frequently damaged somebody close to them, had a history of additional unselective or random violent assaults. Indeed, over half of them had a record of at least one criminal arrest for violence against another person.

Of the prisoners initially surveyed, approximately one-half had a documented history (either before or after imprisonment) of violent assaults against other individuals. Of this group of some 400 individuals we are concerned with the results of detailed examination in 80.

Within the patient group, about one-half had symptoms suggestive of epilepticlike phenomena—including altered states of consciousness, warning states preceding the attack, and postattack sleep, drowsiness, and/or lassitude. In spite of this, only 10 showed traditional temporal lobe epilepsy, 7 of whom had previously been diagnosed as having the disorder.

The incidence of epilepticlike phenomena in the prison group was, like the incidence in our hospital patients, about 50 per cent. And what is more interesting, there were 38 prisoners of the total, with an obvious and known history of epilepsy—an incidence of more than 10 times that which one would expect to find in the general population.

One-third of the 83 hospital patients showed abnormal brain waves—that is, three times the number expected in the general population.* The prison population showed a 50 per cent incidence of abnormal brain waves. It is important to remember, however, that this kind of uncontrolled data must be interpreted with extreme caution. Many in both groups, because of their violence, had suffered numerous head injuries as adults, thus abnormal brain waves may be a result of, rather than a contributor to, their violent behavior. Indeed, over three-quarters of both patients and prisoners had histories of significant periods of unconsciousness from injury or disease.

It is worth noting that in addition to having brought themselves to our attention, more than three-quarters of the hospital patients had previously sought the aid of a psychiatrist or a physician because of symptoms of impulsive violence. A further measure of their concern about their violent behavior is that well over half had made a serious attempt at suicide. Nearly half the hospital patients also had a history of bed wetting past the age of 7; one-fourth a history of fire setting as children; and one-half a history of cruelty to animals.

It is socially significant to note that 55 of the out-patient individuals owned a gun or other lethal weapons, which most of them had used against another individual at least once. Even more striking is the fact that 55, all of whom had licenses to drive a car, volunteered the information that they often used their automobiles to relieve tension, work-out aggression, or as a weapon directed against other people. Most of these 55 individuals freely admitted that they were dangerous drivers.

This comparison of our self-referred patients asking for help with their violent impulses and a series of violent prisoners indicates the symptoms of impulse dyscontrol are almost

* See *Appendix* on p. 136.

identical in the two groups. The reason why the prisoners are in jail and the patients are free (even though 8 of them had committed homicide) seems to be due to factors other than violence itself. The prisoners have a history of criminal behavior other than assaultive or violent behavior, and some were arrested by the police for nonviolent criminal acts. In other cases, violent propensities became evident only in prison.

Thus the dyscontrol syndrome as defined in this chapter is our attempt to point out the important elements in the history of individuals who may be prone to repeated attacks of violence. Some but not all of this group will have structural or functional brain disease. The important thing to remember is that a thorough examination of brain function is necessary in every individual with this characteristic history. It is necessary to identify those people with malfunctioning brains first because their behavior is potentially treatable and their violence can be prevented. Furthermore, it is only by the careful and repeated study of the people in this group that we are going to get the new information that we so desperately need for better neurological and psychiatric tests, and for more exact and rapid identification of the violence-prone individual.

REFERENCES

Bach-y-Rita, G., and Lion, J. Pathological intoxication. Paper presented at the Boston Society of Neurology and Psychiatry. May, 1968.

Blum, R. H. Mind Altering Drugs and Dangerous Behavior: Dangerous Drugs. *Task Force Report: Narcotics and Drug Abuse,* The President's Commission on Law Enforcement and Administration of Justice. Washington, D.C., U.S. Govt. Printing Office, 1967.

Crancer, A., Jr., and McMurray, L. Accident and violation rates of Washington's medically restricted drivers. *JAMA. 205:*272–276, 1968.

Duffy, C. T., with Hirshberg, A. *Sex and Crime.* New York, Doubleday, 1965.

Ervin, F. R., Delgado, J. M. R., Mark, V. M. and Sweet, W. H. Rage: A Para-epileptic phenomenon? Paper presented before the American Epileptic Society, Denver, Colo., November 1968.

Ervin, F. R. The Biology of Individual Violence: A Staff Report to the National Commission on the Causes and Prevention of Violence, No. 13. Washington, D.C., U.S. Govt. Printing Office, December, 1969.

Fenton, G. W., and Udwin, E. L. Homicide, Temporal lobe epilepsy and depression: A case report. *Brit. J. Psychiat. 111:*304–306, 1965.

Gibbs, F. A., Gibbs, E. L., and Lennox, W. G. Epilepsy: A paroxsymal cerebral dysrythmia. *Brain 60:*377–388, 1937.

Gibbs, F. A. Abnormal electrical activity in the temporal regions and its relationship to abnormalities of behavior. *Res. Pub. Ass. Nerv. Ment. Dis. 26:*278, 1956.

Gibbs, F. A. Clinical correlates of 14 and 6 per second positive spikes. *EEG Clin. Neurophiol. 8:*149, 1956.

Glaser, G. H., Newman, R. J., and Schafer, R. "Interictal Psychosis in Psychomotor-Temporal Lobe Epilepsy: An EEG Psychological Study." In: *EEG and Behavior* (G. H. Glaser, ed.). New York, Basic Books, pp. 345–365, 1963.

Hornia, A. Does epilepsy mean higher susceptibility to traffic accidents? *Acta Psychiat. Neurol. Scand. (Suppl.), 150,* 36:210–212, 1961.

Jonas, A. D. *Ictal and Subictal Neurosis: Diagnosis and Treatment.* Springfield, Ill., Thomas, 1965.

Lennox-Buchthal, M., Buchthal, F., and Rosenfalck, P. Correlation of electroencephalographic findings with crash rate of military jet pilots. *Epilepsia 1:*366–372, 1960.

Levy, S., and Kennard, M. A. Study of electroencephalogram as related to personality structure in group of inmates of state penitentiary. *Amer. J. Psychiat. 109:*832–839, 1953.

Lion, J. R., Bach-y-Rita, G., and Ervin, F. R. The self-referred violent patient. *JAMA 205:*503–505, 1968.

Lion, J. R., Bach-y-Rita, G., and Ervin, F. R. Teaching the violent to recognize themselves. *JAMA, 206:*2221–2222, 1968.

Lion, J. R., Bach-y-Rita, G., and Ervin, F. R. Violent patients in the Emergency Room. *Amer. J. Psychiat. 125:*12, 1969.

Loomis, S. D. EEG abnormalities as a correlate of behavior in adolescent male delinquents. *Amer. J. Psychiat. 121:*1003–1006, 1965.

MacDonald, J. M. *The Murderer and His Victim.* Springfield, Ill., Thomas, 1961.

MacDonald, J. M. Suicide and homocide by automobile. *Amer. J. Psychiat. 121:*366–370, 1964.

Mark, V. H., Ervin, F. R., Geschwind, N., Solomon, P., and Sweet, W. H. The neurology of behavior: Its application to human violence. *Med. Opin. Rev. 4:*26–31, 1968.

Mark, V. H., Ervin, F. R., Sweet, W. H., Solomon, P., and Geschwind, N. Brain Disease and Violent Behavior. In: *Neuro-ophthalmology, vol. IV, Ch. 20.* St. Louis, Mosby, 1968, pp. 282–287.

Mark, V. H., and Ervin, F. R. Is there a need to evaluate the individuals producing human violence? *Psychiat. Opinion 5:*32–34, 1968.

Menninger, K. A. *The Vital Balance.* New York, Viking, 1963.

Monroe, R. R. *Behavioral Disorders*. Cambridge, Mass., Harvard Univ. Press. 1970.

Podolsky, E. The epileptic murderer. *Medico-Legal J. 30:*176–179, 1962.

Satten, J., Menninger, K., Rosen, I., and Mayman, M. Murder without apparent motive: A study in personality disorganization. *Amer. J. Psychiat. 117:*48–53, 1960.

Schwade, E. D., and Geiger, S. G. Severe behavior disorders with abnormal electroencephalograms. *Dis. Nerv. System 21:*616–620, 1960.

Selzer, M. L., and Weiss, S. Alcoholism and traffic fatalities: study in futility. *Amer. J. Psychiat. 122:*762–767, 1966.

Shupe, L. M. Alcohol and crime. J. Crim. Law, Criminol. Polit. Sci. *44:*661–664, 1954.

Silverman, D. EEG and criminals. *Arch. Neurol. Psychiat. 52:*38–42, 1944.

Stafford-Clark, D., and Taylor, F. H. Clinical and electroencephalographic studies of prisoners charged with murder. *J. Neurol. Neurosurg. Psychiat. 12:*325–330, 1949.

Storr, A. *On Human Aggression,* New York, Atheneum, 1968.

Small, J. G. The organic dimension of crime. *Arch. Gen. Psychiat. 15:*82–89, 1966.

Task Force Report. Drunkenness. The President's Commission on Law Enforcement and Administration of Justice. Washington, D.C., U.S. Govt. Printing Office, 1967.

Treffert, D. A. The psychiatric patient with an EEG temporal lobe focus. *Amer. J. Psychiat. 120:*765–771, 1964.

United States Department of Health, Education, and Welfare: Report of the Secretary's Advisory Committee on Traffic Safety. Washington, D.C., U.S. Govt. Printing Office, February 29, 1968.

Valles, J. *From Social Drinking to Alcoholism*. Dallas, Texas, Tane Press, 1969, p. 54.

West, D. J. *Murder Followed by Suicide*. Cambridge, Mass., Harvard Univ. Press. 1966.

Willett, T. C. *Criminal on the Road.* London, Havistock, 1964.

Winkler, G. E., and Kove, S. S. Implications of electroencephalographic abnormalities in homicide cases. *Neuropsychiat. 3:*322–330, 1962.

Wolfgang, M. E., and Strohm, R. B. The relationship between alcohol and criminal homicide. *Quart. J. Stud. Alcohol 17:*411–425, 1956.

Wolfgang, M. E. Patterns in Criminal Homicide. Philadelphia, Univ. of Pennsylvania Press, 1958.

Wolfgang, M. E., and Ferracuti, F. *The Subculture of Violence*. London, Tavistock, 1967.

Wolfgang, M. E. (ed.). *Studies in Homicide.* New York, Harper & Row, 1967.

Task Force Report. Narcotics and Drugs. The President's Commission on Law Enforcement and Administration of Justice. Washington, D.C., U.S. Govt. Printing Office, 1967.

Waller, J. A. Medical impairment and highway crashes. *JAMA* *208*:2293–2296, 1969.

Williams, D. Neural factors related to habitual aggression: Considerations of differences between those habitual aggressives and others who have committed crimes of violence. *Brain* 92 (pt. 3): 503–520, 1969.

Appendix

There have been attempts made to conduct a survey of violent individuals by means of (EEG) brain wave recordings, and there is a voluminous literature linking electroencephalographic changes with criminal behavior. Included among the population studied are such diverse groups as "psychopaths" and "felons." Several such studies bear comment. In England, Stafford-Clark and Taylor analyzed the EEGs of 64 murderers, dividing them on the basis of clinical history into categories such as "incidental," "motiveless," "sexual," and "schizo-epileptic." The authors report incidences of abnormal findings for the various groups and an overall incidence of 70 per cent nonspecific abnormal EEGs in criminals whose crimes appeared to be "motiveless." Gibbens investigated EEGs of 72 "severe psychopaths" and 59 controls, reporting a higher incidence of abnormal tracings in the former. In America, Winkler studied 55 patients with "homicidal actions" and found 24 per cent of them to have abnormal brain waves. Silverman divides a prison population into no less than nine classifications: including such labels as "hostile," "hedonistic," "homosexual," "psychotic," etc. Among 411 prisoners, 75 per cent of "psychopathic" criminals had borderline or abnormal EEGs. Levy found 15 per cent abnormal EEGs in both violent and nonviolent murderers. Gibbs, studying EEG tracings in 132 diverse prisoners and 1168 controls composed of college-age normal volunteers, found a 20 per cent incidence of abnormalities in both groups when data were corrected for age.

The diversity of results in studies mentioned above illustrates the extreme variability in EEG techniques, definition of criminal behavior and interpretation, use of control groups, and correction of data for age. Criteria of EEG abnormality are not given by Levy, Gibbens, or Winkler, although sample tracings are illustrated in the last two studies. Similarly, clinical criteria for the labeling of populations as "severe psychopaths" or "incidental" are not identified in reports by Stafford-Clark, but are labeled as "ordinary prisoners" (in contrast to murderers), while Gibbs and Silverman have used normal volunteer populations. EEG interpretation is a subject neglected in the literature and there is an obvious need for double-blind techniques in evaluating tracings from subject and control populations. Finally, sleep EEGs are not included in evaluations by authors Levy, Stafford-Clark, Gibbens, and Silverman.

A recent study by Small attempts to elucidate organic factors in 100 patients convicted of various felonies. Of this sample, 33 per cent showed EEG abnormalities, while 77 per cent displayed indication of organic dysfunction (seizure history, head injury, neurological signs, and "organicity" in psychological examination). All were considered to be mentally ill. This study illustrates the need for thorough neurologic and psychiatric evaluation of criminal patients, and shows that single, isolated screening EEGs alone are misleading in identifying underlying pathology. Not only is a single EEG insufficient evidence for the diagnosis of a seizure disorder, but psychiatric illness can also coexist with seizure patterns.

Of more value is the recent report by Williams, correlating brain wave changes in prisoners with repetitive aggressive behavior as contrasted to prisoners with a single violent episode. Williams has attempted to eliminate patients from both groups with obvious brain dysfunction or head injury and his distinguished career in interpreting brain waves gives the study greater credibility. The prisoners with repetitive assaultive behavior had a significantly higher percentage of abnormal EEGs than did those whose crime was a single act.

Chapter 10

The Either/Or Philosophy

Nothing is so firmly believed as what we least know.

Montaigne

Essays, Book I, Chapter 31

Human behavior, violent or peaceful, is always the product of *brain-environment* interaction. Neither of these two influences can solely determine behavior; but many sociologists and some neurologists talk and act as if this were so. This dualistic view, which states that behavior is generated *either* by the environment *or* by the brain, impedes any rational approach to the understanding and treatment of violent individuals. And at the present time, it is translated by many sociologists, psychiatrists, psychologists, and public officials to mean that human disorders characterized by dementia, paralysis, and blindness are brain problems—problems to be handled by neurologists. At the same time they insist that people with emotional disturbance or behavior disorders—*including the expression of violence*—have a problem which has been solely determined by faulty environment. Thus they reason that these problems can only be handled by social scientists or social psychiatrists. Further, some of them deny that an alteration in brain function could play a role in these disorders and, in fact, they tend to believe that violent individuals do not require a thorough examination of brain function.

This separation of brain from environment has ancient roots, for "dualism" can be traced back at least to Aristotle. He distinguished between the soul (mind) and the body, and he subdivided the soul into parts: one he considered irrational—that is, "shared by man with all living things and vegetative." The other part was "sometimes irrational and yet in a sense partakes of reason." Aristotle's views became the orthodoxy of the Church, and as such affected the work of investigators interested in the nature of the brain. Dualism was still the accepted point of view in the 17th century, when René Descartes began his ruminations on the nervous system. Descartes was the first man to describe reflex activity; but since he wished to avoid antagonizing the academic and religious establishments, he said that the reflex actions—such as walking, running, and moving the arm—were responsive to the commands of the lower nervous system, and carefully separated them from the "mind," which carried out the process of thinking.

Descartes' opinions, which thus perpetuated Aristotle's dualism, influenced later experimental neurologists, such as Sir Charles Sherrington. Sherrington, whose outstanding experimental work laid the foundation for major present-day concepts about the central nervous system, believed that only the mind was involved in the process of thought, and that this capacity for thought was separate from the function of the brain. In this century it was not until the work of George Eliot Coghill and the brothers Herrick that experimental neurology began to unify the concepts of mind and brain. Coghill was able to show that the developing nervous system in salamander larvae acted as an integrated whole, so that bodily movements were coordinated and the larvae were able to swim and find food while their sense organs and sensory nerves were as yet unformed. As the sensory system did develop, it refined and synchronized the animal's behavior, but it did so on the basis of the integrated pattern already established. It took control of a motor system that was already working in a coordinated and efficient manner.

The more brain scientists have discovered about the brain, the clearer it has become that brain responses and the parallel behavior are not separate events—that is, there is no aspect of human behavior that is supernatural. Once we are aware that thinking is a physical process, Aristotle's "soul" and Descartes' "mind" are no longer useful concepts. Unfortunately, dualism still lives on in the work of those who wish to explain the causes of behavior without taking the brain into account, and hence distinguish environment as a separate factor in generating emotional reactions. We strongly disagree with this point of view. It is our position that once environment is perceived, it is incorporated into the brain. Furthermore, any influence that environment has on behavior is exerted exclusively by the brain.

Obviously the normal performance of complicated acts of human behavior does require the function of many bodily organs besides the brain. Nonetheless, we know that the brain does govern what we do. Meaningful behavior is still possible when someone is blind or deaf; a person whose arms and legs are paralyzed still functions in a complicated and purposeful although limited way; the loss of stomach, gallbladder, and/or large portions of the intestines does not prevent meaningful behavior, and the use of kidney, liver, lung, and heart transplants has proved that the recipient's personality and behavior are not changed as long as these transplants function adequately. The injury or destruction of critical parts of the brain, on the other hand, affects behavior in a most dramatic fashion. A tiny damage to the midbrain, for example, will put an end to all meaningful behavior by producing profound and permanent coma. Heart, lungs, liver, and kidneys may function quite adequately and life may persist for a considerable length of time, but there is no perception or adaptation to the environment.

The brain is unique among body organs in that it does not function exclusively within the confines of the body. Through the retina of the eye, and the nerves that receive and convey sensory perceptions of the world, the brain operates outside the skull, confirming and interacting with the external events as well as those that occur inside the body. It is unique in another way also: it has the capacity, after perceiving these events, to store them for future reference in its own tissue. This process, of course, is what we call memory; and it is an essential part of learning, for past experiences of all kinds play an important role in determining an individual's reaction to current environmental stimuli. To put it another way: past environment in the form of memory, determines to a great extent how we react to our present environment, but memory itself is actually incorporated in brain tissue and thus, information retrieval is a brain process.

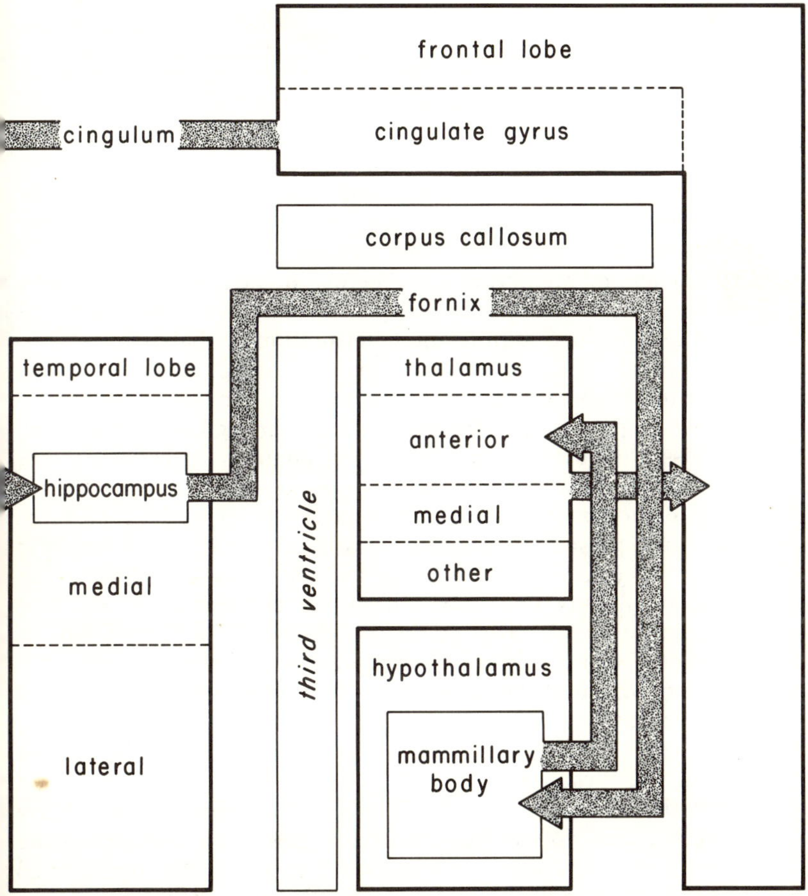

FIG. 38. Major components of the human memory circuit. This schematic diagram of the memory circuit shows that many anatomical structures subserving memory are also important in controlling emotion (see Chapter 2). (This schema is similar to a diagram in the reference by R. G. Ojemann.)

Our past environment, once it is past, is no longer a sociological phenomenon. It is imbedded in our brain and its use is dependent on the function or malfunction of the cerebral tissue.

Major parts of the memory circuit are in the same anatomical location as the limbic brain. The schema in Figure 38, shows the most important of those areas that are involved in the encoding of ongoing environmental stimuli into the memory process. We know that these areas are important for memory because of what happens when they are damaged. If, for example, both hippocampi are injured, a man may literally be unable to remember what happens from one minute to the next. If someone says "good morning" to him and then moves out of his sight for more than 30 seconds, this man will not be able to remember seeing or speaking to the other person when he steps in front of him again. Memories from before the time of injury may remain intact, but the inability to retain recent memory will naturally produce significant deterioration in behavior.

In contrast, lesions or damage to the thalamus may cause profound deficits in the entire memory relationship to the world. The whole personality structure may be involved in such a memory loss with subsequent distressing changes in behavior. For example, a 43-year-old accountant, who suffered a significant brain hemorrhage, became completely disoriented as to time, place, and person. He was awake and alert and able to see and follow objects, and could move both his hands and feet; but he retained only one item out of his cultural past. He kept repeating over and over again the phrase, "The fastest gun in the West," which was all he remembered. He did not recognize his own wife and children when they came to visit him; and to their pathetic attempts to remind him who they were, he could only mumble, "The fastest gun in the West, the fastest gun in the West."

Another aspect of "memory" in the social sense is the ability to retain and follow cultural rules governing behavior. The "rules" for urination, for instance, are culturally determined and rigidly controlled and enforced. We learn them young, and follow them thereafter. Yet a lesion in the brain is able to destroy even this kind of strictly regulated behavior. A case that illustrates this point was that of a 62-year-old bank executive who suffered intractable pain secondary to advanced cancer. Medication did not help him, and the only way to alleviate his pain was to make a destructive lesion in the white matter of his frontal lobe. After he recovered from the operation, he went back to his normal routine as if nothing had happened. He said that he felt well, and he insisted that he and his wife go to an opera opening. He dressed himself immaculately in formal evening attire and walked with his wife from their house to the theater. His conversation was witty and urbane. About half way there, he said, "Excuse me," and in full view of oncoming traffic and pedestrians, he urinated in the street! His brain had lost the use of a basic cultural taboo, and hence some of its capacity to predict the consequences of behavior.

While it is quite true that sensible behavior within the environment depends on brain function, it is also true that the brain functions very poorly in the absence of meaningful environment. In fact, it tends to malfunction under conditions of sensory deprivation or monotony. Furthermore, as we have seen, anatomical development of some segments of the brain depends on environmental stimuli. If a kitten's eyelids are sutured directly after birth and reopened 3 months later, the kitten will be blind because cells in the visual pathways of the brain will have degenerated. On a more complex level, maternal deprivation in newborn monkeys produces profound behavioral changes which persist throughout the monkey's life. These deprived animals have a distinctly inappropriate or exaggerated flight or fight reaction, indicating dysfunction of the brain stem or limbic brain. The brain areas governing sexual activity are also affected by this environmental deprivation: some of these male monkeys engage in homosexual activity, but most of them are unable to complete normal coitus with a receptive female.

The brain and central nervous system always act as a unit in responding to the environment with any kind of behavior, including violence. The involvement of the brain is not the less, therefore, even when some plausible environmental cause precedes a violent action. However, a poorly functioning brain—particularly one with disease or malfunction of the limbic system—is much more apt to be triggered into expressing abnormal behavior by a minimal or inappropriate environmental stimulus than a normal brain. For example, Edna C., the 36-year-old wife of a Baptist clergyman, had had over a 6-year period inappropriate outbursts of rage interspersed with epileptic attacks and associated with a progressive memory loss. A brain wave examination indicated abnormal electrical activity in her temporal region. One afternoon she was being examined by a psychologist, who was testing her memory. Edna grew increasingly frustrated as she realized she could not answer his persistent questions, and finally brought the examination to a close by throwing a pan of water at the psychologist. He began leaving the room, and she hastened his retreat by picking up a bottle of orange soda, swinging it wildly over her head, and hurling it with great force after him. The point here is that she reacted in an inappropriate way to an environmental stimulus; but we could not begin to understand why she assaulted the psychologist if we did not take both his actions and her brain disease into account in assessing her behavior.

In summary, the separation of "mind" from body was the historical idea that nurtured the separation of "environment" from brain. Brain scientists have largely discredited the mind-body dualism; but the environment-brain dualism lives on in the minds and actions of many social scientists and is encoded in our laws. They see behavior and especially violent behavior as being caused only by defects in the environment. Some of them go so far as to admit that the brain may play a significant role in behavior, but many claim it is no good investing time and money in brain research because the brain is too complicated and poorly understood. On the other hand, they predicate their efforts to control violent individuals by rehabilitation or by punishment on the basis that these individuals (*a priori*) have a completely normal brain. That some of these people may have brain disease and are candidates for a combined medical-sociological approach seems to have eluded them. Often, in their isolation from biologists, they fail to realize that every element of environment is intimately connected to brain and brain function, and by ignoring this fact they not only disregard the futility of their solo efforts to treat people with brain injuries, but they pass up the opportunity to study and learn from the brain physiologists new techniques that may be powerful tools of the future for the rehabilitation of violent individuals with normal brains. Thus does the doctrine of separation—the either/or philosophy—continue to exert its pernicious and separatist effect on those of us who are concerned with the diagnosis and treatment of the violent individual.

REFERENCES

Aristotle. The Theory of the Good Life. In: *From Aristotle to Platinius* (T. V. Smith, ed.). Chicago, Univ. Chicago Press, 1934, p. 80.

Aristotle. *De Anima I* (Wallace, trans.).

Coghill, G. E. Correlated anatomical and physiological studies of the growth of the nervous system of Amphibia. *J. Comp. Neurol. 51:*311, 1930.

Collins, G. H., Victor, M., and Adams, R. D. A neuropathological study of Wernicke's disease and Korsakoff's psychosis. *J. Neuropath. Exp. Neurol. 20:*289–291, 1961.

Descartes, R. "Meditations on the First Philosophy." In: *From Descartes to Locke* (T. V. Smith and Marjorie Green, eds.). Chicago, Univ. Chicago Press, 1940, p. 110.

Harlow, H. F. "Development of the Second and Third Affectional Systems in Macaque Monkeys." In: *Research Approaches to Psychiatric Problems: A Symposium* (T. T. Tourlentes, S. L. Pollock, and H. E. Himwich, eds.). New York, Grune & Stratton, pp. 209–229, 1962.

Harlow, H. F. The heterosexual affectional system in monkeys. *Amer. Psychol. 17:*1–9, 1962.

Harlow, H. F. "The Development of Affectional Patterns in Infant monkeys." In: *Determinants of Infant Behavior* (B. M. Foss, ed.). London, Methuen, pp. 75–88, 1961.

Herrick, C. J. *The Evolution of Human Nature.* Austin, Univ. Texas Press, 1956.

Hubel, D. H. Effects of distortion of sensory imput on the visual system of kittens. *The Physiologist 10:*17–45, 1967.

Ojemann, R. G. Correlations between specific human brain lesions and memory changes: A critical survey of the literature. *Neuro-sci. Res. Prog. Bul. 4* (Suppl.): 1–70, 1966.

Sherrington, C. "Forward" in *Integrative Action of the Nervous System.* Cambridge, Cambridge Univ. Press, 1947.

Chapter 11

The Relation of the Dyscontrol Syndrome to Violence in Our Society

> *[In the state of nature] no arts, no letters, no society and, which is worst of all, continual fear and danger of violent death, and the life of man solitary, poor, nasty, brutish and short.*
>
> ***Thomas Hobbes***
> **Leviathan**

The F.B.I. statistics on violence indicate that in 1968 there were over 14,000 murders, 31,000 rapes, and 288,000 cases of aggravated assault in the United States. This represents a 10 to 15 per cent increase over 1967's figures. There were also an estimated million* cases of assault against infants and children, and 60,000 deaths and 3 million injuries caused by automobile accidents. We cannot pretend to say how much of this mayhem was committed by individuals with abnormalities of the brain, since we have no factual data on this matter one way or the other. What we can say, however, on the basis of both sociological and biological studies, is that seriously violent acts are likely to be carried out by individuals who have given at least some warning of trouble to come. There is considerable evidence to indicate that much of the violence is

* This total is based on figures for 1965.

done by people who have poor impulse control, who have a previous history of violent acts, and who keep repeating their impulsive and violent behavior even when it is obviously in their own interest not to do so.

Whatever the underlying causes for this violence, the fact is that it does exist and its incidence is apparently rising. The best efforts of sociologists, educators, psychologists, social pychiatrists, and public officials along with millions of dollars worth of governmental aid have not been able to reverse this trend or diminish the amount of violence. The question thus arises: Can this violence ever be controlled by the kind of environmental manipulations now being used even if it were done well, or is some additional approach worth trying?

It is relatively easy to see that an environmental approach is not likely to have much effect on the cases we cited to illustrate the dyscontrol syndrome. Tony D. and Theresa L. were not only impulsively violent, they had difficulty in restraining their impulses in all other areas of their lives, too. Nor were they deterred by the knowledge or threat of punishment, because the mechanisms that keep most of us from immediately acting on our impulses were deficient or absent in them. Some of the prisoners we saw were similarly unable to control their behavior, no matter what the circumstances. A notorious and skillful bank robber who successfully eluded capture in three states was picked up while carrying $300,000 because he had, on impulse, decided to steal a car and drive from Las Vegas to Reno. Another prisoner, who had robbed a large jewelry store and was driving away after the robbery, decided that he would jump the stop light at a busy intersection; he had the misfortune to run head on into a police car and subsequently found it difficult to explain what the burglar's tools, gun, and large assortment of valuable jewelry were doing on the front seat of his car. It is impossible with present methods to re-educate or to threaten such people into behaving rationally. They are too easily provoked by environmental stimuli, and too unable to control their inappropriate reactions.

Nonetheless, something must be done. The need for finding some way to curb violence and to identify abnormal and potentially violent individuals grows ever more acute as technological advances in bacteriology and chemistry make it more and more possible for a single abnormal person to kill great numbers of people.

The Texas tower tragedy in Austin, in which Charles Whitman shot 41 people, killing 17, and Richard's Speck's murder of 8 nurses in Chicago, are examples of preventable public catastrophes. Weeks before committing his crime, Whitman told a psychiatrist of having "forced thoughts" about climbing the tower and killing many students with a rifle. And after he was killed, his postmortem examination showed he had a brain cancer—the kind of cancer that could have been picked up on a routine isotope scan of the brain. Of course, Whitman's life might not have been saved, as the cancer was highly malignant; but if he had been in the hospital under treatment, he certainly would not have been able to carry out his mass murders. Richard Speck, too, had symptoms of serious brain disease. Both he and Whitman had committed acts of senseless brutality before they murdered. If they had been identified as potentially violent men, and treated before it was too late—before they killed, instead of afterwards—they might have been stopped in time to save their victim's lives.

Oswald, the alleged assassin of President Kennedy, is another example of someone about whom eventual murders could have been predicted. He had a history of repeated episodes of uncontrolled impulsive assaultive behavior before he attempted to assassinate General Walker or kill Officer Tippitt. He was involved in a number of street fights and tried to commit suicide by slashing his wrists when he was in Russia. In addition, he beat his wife unmercifully on a number of occasions. Their neighbors noticed that Marina's head, face, and neck were often severely bruised, and were afraid that one day he would kill her.

These well-publicized and socially important tragedies simply underscore the need for a program that will help us understand and prevent violence. The present methods—which depend upon changing only environmental factors—have proved inadequate; and, in persons whose violence is related to brain dysfunction, they will undoubtedly continue to be inadequate.

Even though sociological and environmental approaches to control violent behavior have failed to produce much in the way of constructive results, they should not be lightly dismissed, and we do not mean to downgrade the obvious importance of social or environmental influences on the brain and behavior. Workers in the field of sociology, criminology, and social anthropology have produced an extensive literature on the subject of human violence. Without covering this field in any detail, we will mention and describe several of the theories that have been formulated to explain the causes of human violence.

One of these is the culture-conflict hypothesis of Thorsten Sellen. This conflict has been described as the natural outgrowth of the process of social differentiation, which, in turn, produces an infinity of social groupings, each with its own definitions of like situations, its own interpretations of social relations, and its own ignorance or misunderstanding of the social values of other groups. Sellen and his followers have suggested that the transformation of a culture from a well-integrated, homogeneous one to a disintegrated type is accompanied by an increase in conflict situations. If this theory had universal applicability, an extremely homogeneous society would be a peaceful one, but the example of Hitlerian Germany suggests that the concept must have exceptions. That country was both homogeneous and well-integrated and yet was infamous for mass murder and brutality.

Some scientists have developed useful models of violent behavior on the basis of individual and group frustrations, with subsequent aggressive behavior. While it is certainly true that frustrating environmental situations play a genuine role in generating violent behavior, individuals vary greatly in their tolerance to frustrating situations. Furthermore, the relation of frustration to violence, in any given individual, is by no means constant. Clearly, we would emphasize the role of the individual's threshold for violent action in defining the outcome of the frustration experience. The applicability of this model to group behavior is another matter.

Cloward and Ohlin, as well as Wolfgang and Ferracuti contend that the form of social violence is determined by a subcultural nominative system. They suggest that a predisposition to violence is transmitted by child-raising practices and peer group relationships in certain segments of the population; their focus is on the urban male in lower socioeconomic groups. While differing subculture norms for acceptable expressions of emotion account for much diversity in our pluralistic society, we would predict that within a given subculture, those individuals most likely to commit personal violence, are those with poor impulse control of the kind we have described.

Yablonsky and others have studied the violent behavior of juvenile urban gangs. In some ways these gangs empitomize certain urban subcultures, but it is difficult to estimate the contribution of juvenile gangs to the total picture of violent behavior. For example, in 1963, there were 1,131 gang incidents in New York City (as recorded by Chwast and Seller). However, these many incidents, each involving a number of participants, resulted in the slaying of "only" 12 people. While the slaying of anyone is a great tragedy, it is difficult to accept this phenomenon as a major source of homicide in New York City.

Recently the subculture theories have been criticized by Endleman. He states:

> Research and theory which assume that the subculture of the poor generates violent behavior reflect on the subculture bias of the behavioral scientist who is developing the theory. The middle-class-oriented behavioral scientist abhors racial theories. As a result, he generally tends to shun theories based on physiology. Having convinced himself that he has successfully removed all vestiges of racism from his formulations, the theorist retains his prejudices, imputing characteristics to a population he does not fully understand while denying that these characteristics exist within his own group. Some criminologists are coming to the conclusion that the case for subcultural violence is overstated. (From *Violence in the Streets* edited by Shalom Endleman. Copyright © 1968 by Shalom Endleman.)

One might summarize the sociological approaches by saying that social disintegration, frustrations and aggressions, and the subcultural norms of violence all play a part in generating violent behavior. There seems, however, to be no general agreement among sociologists or cultural anthropologists on the relative importance of these mechanisms; nor have these theories led, as yet, to definitive programs which have reduced the incidence of the violent behavior in our society.

Frederick Wertham among others has emphasized the role of mass media and particularly television in changing the climate of public opinion and the level of general acceptance of violent behavior. This is an appealing hypothesis, but it is difficult to get objective evidence or to devise experimental situations that give a convincing formulation of the effect of mass media on human behavior. Bandura and his associates have studied the effect of aggressive models (movies and cartoons of violence) on 48 boys and 48 girls enrolled in the Stanford University Nursery School. They found that a significant percentage of their subject would copy what they had seen if the tools were available in applying "aggression" to inanimate objects. The experiment still left unanswered the question as to whether these subjects would have engaged in personal violence had they had the opportunity to do so.

Studies are being undertaken which should contribute to answering this question. Clearly the thousands of hours of exposure to television experienced by the average maturing brain must be reflected in its final structure. However, if television were the principle determinant of violence it would be difficult to explain the disparity in the aggravated assault rates (almost 8 to 1) when one compares Boston and Montreal, as these cities are both saturated with the same television programs. This does not mean that a relationship between television violence and actual violence does not exist; it simply means that we cannot define it at the present time.

The obvious importance and social significance of group violence is hampered by the difficulties in critically analyzing this phenomenon. Wars are the most devastating sort of group violence, since they produce the greatest number of deaths, injuries, and most widespread destruction of property. In an army of national conscripts, chosen by the lottery method, focal brain disease probably poses a minor problem *except in those individuals who lose control of themselves* under the stress of battle and kill their own comrades or innocent civilians.

Revolutions, revolts, and riots provide an interesting borderline area of study. The anatomy of the urban riot has been lucidly dissected by John Spiegel, while Ohlin has thoroughly studied the phenomenon of prison riots.

One of the outstanding features of the widespread urban riots that have recently swept through the United States is the relatively small amount of personal violence committed compared to the large number of people taking part in the riot. In the Watts community of 330,000 people, there were about 10,000 rioters; 37 people were killed, and 118 were wounded by gun fire. Some of these people were killed by police and National Guard troops and some were killed when they were unwittingly left behind in burning buildings. It is our opinion that the riot atmosphere represents a powerful environmental influence on all those people taking part in the riot. The fact that so few people were killed or injured in these riots makes us believe that unusually strong control mechanisms were operating both in the individual rioters and in the police and National Guard troops who sought to keep the riot under control. It would be particularly interesting under these circumstances to examine in detail those individuals who did cause serious injury or death—be they rioters or members of the police and National Guard.

It is important to keep in mind that each individual taking part in a riot has a unique life experience stored in his brain. Furthermore, each individual receives unique visual, auditory, cutaneous, olfactory, and gustatory cues which are transmitted to his brain for the integration and synthesis that result in the vocalizations and muscular movements of human behavior. This is not to deny the tremendous homogenizing influence that a group has on any individual taking part in group activity. Nevertheless, each individual is responsible for his own behavior; that this behavior may blend perfectly into the group activity is a tribute to the flexibility and adaptability of the central nervous system. It does not mean that an individual's brain has ceased to function, nor does it mean that his individual behavior can be ignored.

The increase in both group and individual domestic violence has brought two kinds of responses from an afflicted society. One approach concentrates on the rigid enforcement of "law and order." This phrase has often been a euphemism for the suppression of public demonstrations and protests. It brings with it the specter of an authoritarian police state. The other approach to the control of violence calls for the dissolution of the slums, the abolition of poverty, and the correction of social injustices—all vitally necessary goals. Up to this time neither of these approaches in their piecemeal application has resulted in an effective reduction of violent behavior. But both of these approaches have one thing in common: they ignore the individual and his brain.

Finally, we should like to emphasize that—in spite of our apparent criticism of our sociologically oriented colleagues—we realize that these professionals are working in a difficult and complex field. However, they should not have to labor alone. With new technological skills and equipment, the brain scientists and clinicians can give them some significant help. Together the two disciplines can shoulder the public burden that violence causes.

REFERENCES

Altman, J., and Ziporyn, M. C. *Born to Raise Hell.* New York, Grove Press, 1967.

Bandura, A., Ross, D., and Ross, S. A. Imitation of film-mediated aggressive models. *J Abnorm. Soc. Psychol. 66:*3–11, 1963.

Carthy, J. D., and Ebling, F. J. (eds.). *The Natural History of Agression.* New York, Academic Press, 1964.

Cloward, R. A. "Social Control in the Prisons." In: *Theoretical Studies of the Social Organization of the Prison, Bulletin #15,* March 1960.

Cloward, R. A., and Ohlin, L. E. *Delinquency and Opportunity.* Glencoe, Ill., The Free Press, 1960.

Cohen, J., and Murphy, W. S. *Burn, Baby, Burn.* New York, Avon Books, 1966.

Endleman, S. (ed.) *Violence in the Streets,* Chicago, Quadrangle Books, 1968.

Ford, G. R., and Stiles, J. R. *Portrait of an Assassin.* New York, Ballentine Books, 1965.

Gibbs, F. A., Bagchi, B. K., and Bloomberg, W. EEG study of criminals. *Amer. J. Psychiat. 102:*294–298, 1945.

Glueck, S., and Glueck, E. *Predicting Delinquency and Crime.* Cambridge, Mass., Harvard Univ. Press, 1959.

Goldensohn, E. S. EEG and Ictal and Postictal Behavior. In: *EEG and Behavior* (G. H. Glaser, ed.). New York, Basic Books, pp. 293–314, 1963.

Graham, H. D., and Gurr, T. R. *Violence in America: Historical and Comparative Perspectives.* New York, Bantam Books, 1969.

Helfer, R. E., and Kempe, C. H. (eds.) *The Battered Child.* Chicago, Univ. of Chicago Press, 1968.

Johnson, N., Savitz, L. and Wolfgang, M. E. (eds.) *The Sociology of Punishment and Correction.* New York, Wiley, 1962.

Levy, S., and Kennard, M. A. Study of electroencephalogram as related to personality structure in group of inmates of state penitentiary. *Amer. J. Psychiat. 109:*832–839, 1953.

Mark, V. H., and Ervin, F. R. Is there a need to evaluate the individuals producing human violence? *Psychiat. Opinion 5:*32–34, 1968.

Mark, V. H., Ervin, F. R., Sweet, W. H., Solomon, P., and Geschwind, N. "Brain Disease and Violent Behavior." In: *Neuro-opthalmology,* vol. IV. St. Louis, Mosby, pp. 282–287, 1968.

Mark, V. H., Ervin, F. R., Geschwind, N., Solomon, P., and Sweet, W. H. The neurology of behavior: Its application to human violence. *Med. Opin. Rev. 4:*26–31, 1968.

Masotti, L. H., and Corsi, J. R. *Shoot-out in Cleveland: Black Militants and the Police: July 23, 1968*. New York, Bantam Books, 1969.

Menninger, K. *The Crime of Punishment*. New York, Viking Press, 1969.

Silverman, D. EEG and criminals. *Arch. Neurol. Psychiat.* *52:*38–42, 1944.

Small, J .G. The organic dimension of crime. *Arch. Gen. Psychiat.* *15:*82–89, 1966.

Spiegel, J. P. Race relations and violence—a social psychiatric perspective. Presented before the Association for Research in Nervous and Mental Diseases, New York, Dec. 1, 1967.

Spiegel, J. P. Psychosocial factors in riots—old and new. *Amer. J. Psychiat.* *125:*281–285, 1968.

Spiegel, J. P. The tradition of violence in our society. *Washington Star* Oct. 13, 1968.

Spiegel, J. P. "The Social and Psychological Dynamics of Militant Negro Activism: A preliminary Report." In: *The Dynamics of Dissent,* vol. XIII (J. H. Masserman, (ed.). New York, Grune & Stratton, pp. 136–157, 1968.

Stafford-Clark., D. and Taylor, F. H. Clinical and electroencephalographic studies of prisoners charged with murder. *J. Neurol. Neurosurg. Psychiat.* *12:*325–330, 1949.

Sweet, W. H. (Member of Gov. Connelley's Blue Ribbon Committee). On the Whitman case. Personal communication to the authors, 1968.

Walker, D. *Rights in Conflict: "The Chicago Police Riot."* New York, The New American Library, 1968.

Wertham, F. *A Sign for Cain*. New York, Macmillan, 1966.

Wertham, F. *The Show of Violence*. New York, Doubleday, 1949.

Winkler, G. E., and Kove, S. S. Implications of electroencephalographic abnormalities in homicide cases. *Neuropsychiat.* *3:*322–330, 1962.

Wolfgang, M. E. *Patterns in Criminal Homicide*. Philadelphia, Univ. of Pennsylvania Press, 1958.

Wolfgang, M. E., and Ferracuti, F. *The Subculture of Violence*. London, Tavistock, 1967.

Wolfgang, M. E. (ed.) *Studies in Homicide*. New York, Harper & Row, 1967.

World Almanac, 1969.

Yablonsky, L. The violent gang. *Commentary*, *30:*125–130, 1960.

Chapter 12

Violence Prevention

I established law and justice in the land.

The Code of Hammurabi

Chiefs, who no more in bloody fights engage.

Homer

Iliad, Book III

Happy be he who could learn the causes of things and who put beneath his feet all fears.

Virgil

Georgics, I, Line 490

The problem that modern biological and social scientists have in trying to deal with violence is much like the problem that 19th century neurologists and psychiatrists had with "insanity" —learning enough about its causes and natural history to be able to assess individual cases and treat each patient properly. In the 19th century the insane asylums were full of people lumped together as "crazy," but who in reality had many different diseases. Some actually had pellagra. Once doctors could recognize vitamin deficiencies, and know how to prevent and treat them, people no longer developed pellagra-related symptoms of mental illness. Others were suffering from the late stages of syphillis, and still others from undiscovered brain tumors; both conditions became accessible to diagnosis and treatment, thereby shrinking the "crazy" category still further. In short, the more psychiatrists and neurologists learned about the various causes of "insanity," the more effectively were they able to differentiate between mental conditions that appeared to be the same, but, because they had different causes, required very different methods of treatment.

We are in the same state today vis-à-vis violence: we need to find out more about the condition and learn how to sort out its different causes, so that we can decide which are the most important biological and/or social factors in each individual case, and then treat each patient appropriately.

In our view, the best way to go about gathering the information we so desperately need about violence is to start with a sociobiological study of violent persons. This study must be aimed at (1) establishing the physical and social causes for such behavior; (2) developing reliable early-warning tests for violence; (3) assessing presently available methods of treatment, including medical and surgical techniques, as well as behavioral therapies; and (4) establishing community facilities to help violent persons—facilities that also might be used for medical and sociological studies.

This kind of study is a big job and we face it with inadequate tools. The tool we need the most is a satisfactory method of predicting a given individual's threshold for violent acts. That is, we should develop tests for limbic brain function and dysfunction. This development, in turn, will be dependent upon thorough-going investigations of violent individuals who are known to have disease of the limbic brain.

Two kinds of facilities are necessary for any such investigation. One is a place to house the individuals being studied; the other is a medical center staffed with specialists in the field of neurology, psychiatry, neurosurgery, psychology, and genetics. Of necessity, these two institutions should coexist—as they do *not* today—and be set up so that the safety of the community is not jeopardized by the violent patients. This means a building with a particular kind of physical construction, and a staff of physicians, nurses, and attendants who are capable of dealing with the violent behavior of the inmates. Hopefully, this structure would abut or be on the campus of a major university medical center, as this kind of institution is the only one likely to have either specialists and/or physical facilities to carry out complex brain examinations.

The team that studies violent individuals should include not only brain scientists and clinicians, but also social scientists, criminologists, legal experts, cytogeneticists, and specialists in public health. The studies, to be made on each person with a history of violence, should include:

1. A thorough psychiatric examination
2. A complete social history
3. An exacting neurological and general medical examination
4. The appropriate laboratory examinations—including the multiple recording of brain waves, x-ray examination of the head, visual field examinations, special hearing tests, and (if indicated) isotopic brain scans and special x-ray films of the brain itself
5. Psychological examinations, which should include not only the use of techniques for personality assessment but also special tests for brain damage
6. A genetic evaluation, which should include chromosomal analysis, anthropometric measurements (such as fingerprints), an assay of reproductive function, an electrocardiogram, a test of intellectual performance, and a thorough investigation of the family history for instances of mental illness or impairment, infertility or fetal loss, congenital deformities, tumors, and autoimmune disease.

Only time will tell which of these tests will be most valuable in predicting or diagnosing the thresholds for individual violence.

Ideally, this kind of study would be made on two groups: individuals self-referred to the general hospital because of inability to control destructive impulses; and individuals who appear before the courts who have committed violent antisocial acts. After a statistically significant number of individuals in each of these groups has been examined, the data could be compared either to a control group of the brothers and sisters of the hospitalized individuals, or to a control group of other hospital patients admitted for routine matters and matched for age, sex, religion, and socioeconomic factors.

Even more important than applying conventional statistical

methods would be quantitatively assessing the concurrence of the various abnormal factors discovered from the group of patients with episodic violence. It would be necessary to isolate a small population, perhaps 10 to 20 individuals in each group, with a concentration of chromosomal, electrophysiological, psychological, and neurological abnormalities. The testing or development of additional methods of measurement could be done on these smaller samples, and it might even be possible to explore the interaction of the various pertinent variables in producing the violent act.

We have already suggested in Chapter 7 the lines of investigation to be pursued in individuals with both temporal lobe epilepsy and uncontrollable violent behavior. These particular individuals, with implanted brain electrodes, offer an unusual opportunity to assess abnormalities in limbic brain function, and also represent the best chance we have to find out how to detect these abnormalities. We might, for instance, find out if changes in the brain's electrical activity could be correlated with changes in plasma or urine hormone levels; or if there might be a valid correlation with psychological test scores. It is possible that an as yet unperceived relationship might emerge from such studies that would give us a simple test to help predict accurately whether a given person has a dangerously low threshold for impulsive violence.

If detecting a potentially violent individual is the first order of business for meaningful investigation, the second is to improve our treatment methods. This could well start with a reevaluation of the kinds of psychotherapy given to violent patients. As certain forms of conditioning (i.e., conditional reflex therapy—à la Pavlov) have been shown to improve or alleviate special kinds of temporal lobe epilepsy, applications of improved techniques in behavior therapy might have important consequences for the psychotherapeutic treatment of impulse disorders.

The recent pharmacologic advances in anticonvulsants and tranquilizers presage not the end but the beginning of a psychopharmacological revolution. Many new and important chemical agents and drugs will be added to our armamentarium for the treatment of impulsive and violent behavior. But even with these new psychotherapeutic and medicinal tools, some people with brain disease may still require surgical treatment for the control of violence. How can we improve our surgical operations? By making smaller and more precise lesions within the brain? By using electrical stimulation as we did with Thomas R. instead of making destructive brain lesions? Perhaps a prolonged therapeutic effect can be obtained by the introduction of chemical agents into focal areas of the brain to produce chronic chemical stimulation over a long period of time.

We have described our hopes for the newer techniques in the diagnosis and treatment of violent patients. All these matters, however, are tasks for clinicians and investigators who are primarily interested in individuals rather than in groups. It is beyond the scope of this book and, in fact, our competence, to tell specialists in group behavior how to study and influence the prevailing moods in our society that make up the framework of social interaction. But we should like to point out that as long as senseless killings and brutality are acceptable events in our cities, on our highways, and in our foreign relations, then identifying any violent individual as unique will continue to be very difficult indeed. How, in fact, can society even define what is "abnormal" under these circumstances? Only when our society—through its educational, religious, family, and governmental structures—clearly defines and uniformly reacts to violence as being unacceptable, will we be able to approach the situation in a truly rational way.

The definition of "unacceptable violence" is, of course, a major stumbling block. What is "unacceptable violence"? The "law and order" faction of our society might define any liberal group protest as falling into this category, while protesting groups might label any action of police against demonstrators as "police brutality"—a clear-cut case of "unacceptable violence." Some minority groups have gone even further and, having identified the deprivation of civil rights as a form of violence, have equated this term with physical violence, and justified physically violent retaliation.

Obviously any definition of unacceptable violence, no matter how carefully articulated, is going to be responsive to the judgment of the people participating in or observing a given violent action. But we would agree with Harvard's professor of humanities, Howard Mumford Jones, who states in his monograph (*Violence and Reason*): "the celebration of violence either as an end in itself or as a short-cut to political or social change can only end, unless all history is in error, in the disruption of order and culture."

We would define "acceptable violence" as the controlled minimum necessary action to prevent personal physical injury or wanton destruction of property. This definition would apply equally to police or public authorities as well as to politically activist groups (students, racial, etc.), and all violent acts that did not fit into this category would be "unacceptable." We use our definition as an example rather than as dogma. There might be better definitions that could be more readily applied. The important thing, however, is for such a definition to be formulated, publicized, and accepted, for this is a first step in the orderly and systematic process that must be used in our society if we are to find a method of recognizing potentially violent individuals with a malfunctioning brain.

The human species now dominates the earth. Our greatest danger no longer comes from famine or communicable diseases. Our greatest danger lies in ourselves and in our violent fellow humans. In order to reverse the trend of human violence, we must set certain basic standards of behavior (e.g., "golden rule" or "Ten Commandments") that any individual with a normal brain can follow. In addition, we need to find some way to detect those individuals with brain abnormalities who are unlikely to be able to follow those standards. In other words, we need to develop an "early warning test" of limbic brain function to detect those humans who have a low threshold for impulsive violence, and we need better and more effective methods of treating them once we have found out who they are. Violence is a public health problem, and the major thrust of any program dealing with violence must be toward its prevention—a goal that will make a better and safer world for us all.

REFERENCES

Calder, N. (ed.) *Unless Peace Comes: A Scientific Forecast of New Weapons.* New York, Viking Press, 1968.

Delgado, J. M. R. Action of hormones upon brain excitability. *Proc. 20th Int. Physiol. Congr.* No. 469, 1956.

Delgado, J. M. R. "Pharmacological Modifications of Social Behavior." In: *Pharmacological Analysis of Central Nervous Action* (W. D. M. Paton, ed.). Oxford: Pergamon Press, pp. 265–292, 1962.

Delgado, J. M. R. Intracerebral chemo-stimulation in unanesthetized monkeys (Abst.). *Fed. Proc.* 22:515, 1963.

Folkman, J., and Mark, V. H. Diffusion of anesthetic and other drugs through silicone rubber: Therapeutic implications. *Trans. NY Acad. Sci. 30:*1187–1195, 1968.

Folkman, J., Mark, V. H., Ervin, F. R., Suematsu, K., and Hagiwara, R. Intracerebral gas anesthesia by diffusion through silicon rubber. *Anesthesiology 29:*419–425. 1968.

Freedman, D. X., and Giarman, N. J. "Brain Amines, Electrical Activity, and Behavior." In: *EEG and Behavior* (G. H. Glaser, ed.). New York, Basic Books, pp. 198–243, 1963.

Hanai, T., and Delgado, J. M. R. Microinjections of drugs within the brain of awake monkeys (Abst.). *XXIII Int. Congr. Physiol. Sci.* Tokyo, Sept., 1965.

Huber, G. Die Bedeutung der Neuroradiologie fur die Psychiatrie. *Fortsch. Med. 81:*705–709, 1963.

Jones, H. M. *Violence and Reason: A Book of Essays.* New York, Atheneum, 1969.

Kahn, M. W. Correlates of Rorschach reality adherence in the assessment of murderers who plead insanity. *J. Project. Techn. 31:*44–47, 1967.

Lion, J. R., and Thornton, R. The violent patient: Social and vocational aspects of treatment. Unpublished data.

Mark, V. H., Folkman, J., Ervin, F. R., and Sweet, W. H. Focal brain suppression by means of a silicone rubber chemode. *J. Neurosurg. 30:*195–199, 1969.

Appendix I

Social and Ethical Issues: Brain Surgery in Aggressive Epileptics

Reprinted with permission from Mark, V. H. *The Hastings Center Report,* Vol. 3, No. 1, February, 1973. Institute of Society, Ethics and the Life Sciences, Hastings-on-Hudson, New York.

A little over two years ago Frank Ervin, a psychiatrist, and I, a neurosurgeon, wrote a book called *Violence and the Brain,* detailing the application of brain surgery to problems of violent behavior. The public response to that book underscores with great vividness the fact that the medical issues of neurosurgery are no more interesting or vital than the issues of neurosurgery's *social role.* I would like here to offer some reflections about those social issues.

The most important problem to conjure with, from the standpoint of the sciences of human behavior, is the unfortunate dichotomy in basic approaches to behavior. Certain kinds of behavior (for instance, paralysis, blindness and dementia) were put into the province of *organic neurology.* Physicians working in this field have been increasingly reluctant to examine other kinds of abnormal behavior, even when they are associated with obvious brain abnormalities.

On the other hand, social psychiatrists, sociologists, criminologists, and many psychologists tend to view the other behavioral abnormalities, for instance intractable depressions and aggressive assaultive behavior, as pure reflections of unusual or abnormal environmental stress. They believe that brain function or dysfunction is not an important determinant as far as abnormal behavior is concerned. To them, all human beings function with the same "normal" brains.

Even those few social scientists who admit that brain function might be important in abnormal behavior feel that so little is known about brain function that is useless to spend time and money investigating it.

Now whatever the sociological reasons for this division of labor in the scientific vineyard, any high school student can see that it results in absurd theoretical suppositions. No human behavior whatever, be it normal or abnormal, can be the consequence of the brain alone without the environment. Nor can any behavior, whatever its environmental determinants, take place without the brain freighting its mechanical impulses with emotion and culture. Therefore any thorough investigation of abnormal, violent behavior should look not only to the environment for causes but also to the brain itself.

Yet when President Lyndon Johnson and Milton Eisenhower convened the Commission on Violence, there were over fifty consultants representing various fields of sociology, criminology, history, government, law, social psychiatry, and social psychology, but only two representing the brain!

Let me stress that recognition of the brain in behavior does not entail, as some critics might fear, that all behavior should be controlled through the brain. Rather it is precisely because any behavior, normal or abnormal, *could be* modified through altering the brain, at least in principle, that is it absolutely crucial to make *moral* decisions about the sort appropriate for neurosurgery and other direct brain manipulations. There are important moral issues at stake, for example, in the very definition of a problem as a medical one, for which medical therapy is appropriate. This problem is pressed further when a behavior problem is defined as a neurological one.

My own position regarding the appropriateness of neurosurgery can be illustrated in terms of three alternatives. The first two of these I unequivocally reject:

The first of these positions holds that medical means should be undertaken to improve *any* behavior, wherever possible, be the behavior normal or abnormal. Although neurosurgery is not in a position now to improve normal behavior, some people advocate the use of drugs—amphetamines, for instance—for that purpose. The advantage of this position is that it avoids the obvious difficulties in defining normality. The grave disadvantage is that it makes the medical men authorities on improvement and the good life, which they are not, at least under our present social arrangement. Moral values are social concerns, not medical ones in any presently recognized sense.

A second position holds that any *abnormal* behavior should be treated by whatever medical means are available. Often argued by psychotherapists, this position says that, regardless of any *organic* abnormality, what is undesirable in abnormal behavior is the behavior, not its organic base. The criteria for alteration should refer to the behavior, irrespective of whether the organic base is normal or abnormal. Should an unusual brain abnormality produce a 50 point I.Q. *rise,* no one would suggest ablating it: its behavioral product is desirable. (With regard to neurourgical control of violent behavior, I am *against* the principle that it could be used to treat abnormal behavior when there is no organic abnormality of the brain.)

A third position, then, is that medical procedures like neurosurgery should be used only when behavior is abnormal, and bad, as the result of an abnormality in the brain. As I shall repeat below, violent behavior *not* associated with brain disease should be dealt with politically and socially, not medically.

With this brief positioning of what I take to be support for a very circumscribed domain for neurosurgical procedures, I now want to deal with some common criticisms of neurosurgery. Most of the criticisms either construe neurosurgery to be capable of more than it is, or assume that it would be used in areas I believe to be inappropriate. Like any technological power, neurosurgery can be misused, and setting the limits of its use is more than a medical problem.

Political versus Personal Violence

Implicit in many of the criticisms of the surgical treatment of violent epileptics is the fear that this treatment will be used against political protestors. This fear is based on a semantic confusion about the word "violence." Many activities in our society are called violent. The "establishment" tends to view as violent any protest movement against the war, unfair living conditions, or the prison system. Protestors view the reaction of police and the National Guard as violent. Minority groups have indicated that social or job discrimination is a form of violence.

The kind of violent behavior for which I might approve neurosurgery, however, has a much narrower definition: *personal violent behavior; unwarranted and usually unprovoked acts that directly attempt to, or actually do injure or destroy another person or thing.* And, as I have said, I would not approve neurosurgery even in such cases unless the personal violence could be traced to organic brain disease and could not be treated by non-surgical methods.

Some political psychiatrists have argued that social injustice provokes individual acts of violence which seem "senseless" but which, in reality, are political protests against the social system. As Goebbels showed, political violence of mass proportions can be culled up without counting on people with diseased brains. However, the person whose violence is related to brain disease and is used by a Hitler or Goebbels is a danger to himself and his loved ones, and cannot be counted on to rage only in politically strategic situations. Thus, the morality of preventing such an individual from seeking proper medical diagnosis and care is certainly in question.

Biological Factors in Personal Violence

Many sociologists believe that brain dysfunction does not have a role in such behavioral abnormalities as intractable depression, thought disorders, paranoia, or aggressive assaultive behavior of the sort I am concerned with. In the last case, however, there is *solid* medical evidence to link aggressive behavior to focal brain disease. This behavioral symptom is often present in such clinical disorders as temporal lobe epilepsy, temporal lobe tumors, infections of the brain (such as rabies and post-encephalitic syndromes), and serious brain injuries which affect the under-surfaces of the frontal lobes and the anterior tips of the temporal lobes (usually a transient phenomenon in the last disorder).

The most frequent occurrence of brain dysfunction in violent behavior is in brain poisoning, the most serious and ubiquitous of which is caused by alcohol. Alcohol is a specific brain poison and individuals acutely poisoned with alcohol may have as much dysfunction during the poisoning as would be caused by a brain tumor, infection or injury. The only difference between the former and the latter is that alcohol poisoning is temporary.

The violence in automobile accidents caused by drunk drivers takes a far greater toll than the violence in political protest or repression. A drunk driver suffers from a temporary brain abnormality. Although I certainly do not advocate neurosurgery for the treatment of alcoholism, nor for all kinds of organic brain disease, it is clear that violence is sometimes a function of brain abnormalities, and should be viewed as such.

Racism

In the most *avant garde* circles today the favorite critical epithet is "chauvinist." Neurosurgery seems to draw its critics from a somewhat stodgier class: neurosurgical treatment of violent epileptics has been called "racist."

Speaking to a national group of psychiatric investigators about our approach to the problem of violent behavior, a major professor of psychiatry conceded that the biological–social model of violence and the investigation of brain disease associated with violence had some merit. But he classified our project with the proposal of those psychologists who claim that black people have a constitutionally inferior IQ compared to white people. Admitting that the racial idea might have some merit too, he felt that nevertheless funding and research should not be given to such projects until all possible avenues of social and educational rehabilitation have been exhausted.

It seems to me there are really two issues here. The first concerns the political implications of a theory about violence. One of the functions of a theory is that it tells you where to look to find the phenomenon in question. Does the theory that some violence is caused by brain disease lead us to expect it is a characteristic mainly of black people? Certainly not. On the other hand, the theory that personal violence is caused exclusively by social conditions might very well lead us to look at the black ghettos. The environmental cues to personal violence may very well cluster around racially differentiated areas.

The second issue is whether there is any empirical evidence that organically based personal violence is more common among blacks than whites. In my experience there is no special correlation of violence with race. Domestic personal violence occurs in upper- and middle-class homes as well as in the ghettos. When it occurs in the ghetto, however, it may be more visible, spilling out into the streets from the very pressures of overcrowding. It may very well be that violence in ghettos more often gets reported in police records and other data available to the sociologist. But the perspective of the physician is the emergency room and clinic where the products of violence are immediate. From this perspective, claret is the predominant color, not black or white.

It is my perception that the biological–social model of violence will not concentrate on one race, ethnic group, or other social segment of our population as do the subculture theories of violence. In fact, I feel it is important in cases of violence related to brain disease to study the violent act primarily and to consider the style of violence, which is socially determined, as a secondary phenomenon.

Dangers in a Medical Model of Violence

All sorts of dire predictions have been made about the outcome of brain research directed toward the understanding and treatment of emotional disorders, and especially those related to violent behavior.

Shades of 1984! "The neurosurgeons want to put electrodes in everyone's brain to keep them from protesting!" "They're going to develop a new drug that will completely destroy the will!" "Man's dignity will be shattered and his innate human quality will be destroyed!" These would indeed be serious statements if they were true. But it is important to see just what the issues are.

It is one thing to advocate neurosurgical procedures for certain kinds of violent behavior caused by organic brain disease or dysfunction. It is quite another to advocate them as general methods of behavior control. My own belief is that no form of conditioning, drug therapy, or surgery is necessary or desirable to control normal-brained members of our society, no matter what their political views are or how they express them.

Of course it is true that behavior control techniques developed to be used in a circumscribed sphere might be adapted to widespread and immoral ends by unscrupulous people. No greater lesson is needed than that provided by Nazi Germany.

But interestingly enough, the controls Goebbels used were environmental ones, not direct alterations of the brain. No drugs were needed to seduce the German population. The S.S. storm troopers did not have little electrodes implanted in their limbic systems.

Although Joseph Goebbels might have reduplicated Skinner's experiments in the best conditioning traditions, he did so before, rather than after, the fact. As a clinician living among the German people for two years after the war, I could find nothing in them that would distinguish them from other human beings.

Can one imagine the most advanced brain electrode technology of the future, or even a new and much more sophisticated group of psychic drugs, that could produce a more perfect form of behavior control than that initiated by environmental "natural" factors in the Third Reich?

One of the important factors to emerge from our own research on the relative influence of deep electrical brain stimulation versus environmental "natural" stimuli is the importance, in terms of effectiveness, of the latter. Of course, effective electrical brain stimulation in target areas can produce pronounced behavioral effects. However, even in susceptible individuals with brain disease, the effect of nonconvulsing doses of electrical stimulation can be remarkably altered and suppressed by giving the subject a demanding and attention-absorbing task during electrical brain stimulation.

My thesis that behavior control through the direct manipulation of the brain is not as dangerous for mass abuse as environmental forms of control should not be taken to imply that it has no dangers whatsoever for mass abuse. But the social limitations on who performs neurosurgery or administers drugs, on whom, and for what reasons, ought to be set through public discussion and social decision. My own claim is that the dangers of mass abuse are not sufficient to warrant preventing the very development of the techniques that might have very great therapeutic value for patients with organic brain disease.

Moral Problems in Neurosurgery

If neurosurgery is not much of a danger as a political tool, there still are serious problems with its medical use. I would like to address two of these.

First is the problem of neurological diagnosis. The emphasis I have been placing on the neurological side of the problem of violence ought not be taken out of the context of environmental factors also. Due to the very fundamental problem of specialization in medicine, it is very difficult to maintain a biological–social model of violence in actual practice. The neurologists are in one place and the psychiatrists and social workers are in another.

Yet if the model is worthwhile, treatment of a patient should involve not only his brain but his family, living conditions, job and role in society. It is very important, therefore, to imbed a neurological diagnosis of problems of violence into a larger integrated approach to human behavior. The social forms for this holistic therapy are yet to be worked out, although my own group has tried to include psychiatric and social psychiatric diagnosis along with the neurological.

From my reading of the present situation, however, I believe the greater danger is that the neurological side will be left out. Recently, for example, an airplane hijacker killed one pilot and shot another before he himself was subdued with a blow to the head. Examination of this man afterward revealed he had been a neurological cripple for eleven years, ever since receiving a gunshot wound of the brain. Yet repeated tests, including hours of brainwave examinations, psychological testing, psychiatric and neurological assessment, failed to reveal the tremendous damage that had occurred in this man's emotional center or limbic brain.

The difficulties of diagnosis had their classic but tragic expression in the case of George Gershwin. This talented composer was seen and treated psychiatrically for a long time while a tumor in the limbic system of his brain grew to an unmanageable and untreatable size. The George Gershwin syndrome of the thirties is still being treated in the seventies. Recently eighteen patients were committed to a mental hospital at one of our best university centers who turned out to have tumors of their limbic brains. In some cases, the true nature of this illness was not recognized until the tumor had caused the patient's death.

Second, after the diagnosis of brain disease has been confirmed, *what are the problems of proper consent to treatment?* Does the patient consent to the treatment? Does he know the dangers of the treatment, and how those dangers compare with letting him pass without treatment? What are the wider factors involved in informed consent when the patient is mentally incompetent?*

Usually close members of their families are the sources of consent. But in cases of surgery for violence, I believe the patient and his family should have the assistance of an impartial, noninvolved professional group to determine whether surgery or other forms of treatment should be undertaken. In practical terms, this means that a committee of some sort, composed of physicians, or in some cases, physicians and informed laymen, should be present to monitor the medical, psychiatric, and/or surgical treatment.†

In my own practice, I and my group do not accept patients for treatments who do not want therapy, and we do not believe that the public good or public interest should intrude upon the personal medical model in terms of protecting the public against violent individuals.

Free Will and Behavior Control

Radical critics of the biological–social model of violence often construe human violence to be an expression of free will. In line with this they consider the medical correction of brain disease that would, as a secondary result, stop violent episodes, to have an unnatural and degrading effect on human dignity. As a physician I find this view particularly inappropriate, not because I deny free will, but because I prize the quality of human life.

Many of the patients who come to us with focal brain disease associated with violent behavior are so offended by their own actions

*** Prison inmates suffering from epilepsy should receive only medical treatment; surgical therapy should not be carried out, because of the difficulty in obtaining truly informed consent.**

† In conjunction with Dr. David Allen, we are exploring "consumer advocacy" utilizing a group with religious, legal and community representatives in addition to physicians.

they have attempted suicide. They feel their human dignity has been lost precisely because of uncontrollable behavior patterns they find unnatural and repugnant.

Because our work, and that of other physicians, has indicated a clinical relationship between limbic brain disease, such as temporal lobe epilepsy, and aggressive assaultive behavior, *I believe the correction of that organic condition gives the patient more rather than less, control over his own behavior.* It enhances, and does not diminish, his dignity. It adds to, and does not detract from, his human qualities.

Finally, it is appropriate to return to the specter of a tryrannical government controlling a submissive population through neurosurgery and electrical brain stimulation. Even though this is technically unlikely now, it is a possibility to be conjured with. In the face of this possibility I still have great confidence that the neurological research in behavior control now being done will lead to a better understanding of brain mechanisms, and that when this occurs, *it should be possible for brain scientists to devise techniques for making behavior control of one individual by another more difficult or even impossible.*

In other words, one of the expected benefits of increased brain research will be the creation of new techniques enabling each individual better to control or govern his or her behavior, without unwarranted or unwanted interference by other individuals or devices.

There is already enough knowledge of environmental and psychopharmacological drugs to control a vast segment of our population, without invoking brain surgery or electrical brain stimulation. The great hope of emotional brain research is that it will free us from our present tyrannies and future danges of control. To this end brain scientists need the help of philosophers, ethicists, theologians, social scientists and jurists, working in concert.

Appendix II

Recent Data on Case Histories

Since the publication of this monograph in 1970, important new information linking brain malfunction to abnormal aggression has been reported. Vaernet[1] has performed electroencephalographic recordings and subsequent amygdalotomies in patients who were described as violent psychopaths. Those of his patients with an epileptic-like discharge from their amygdala had a reduction in abnormal aggressivity after the operation. However, with one exception, patients with normal brain wave recordings had no change in their behavior after operation.

Recently, Walker[2] gave the John Hughlings Jackson oration at the Montreal Neurological Institute, reviewing his physiological and surgical findings in temporal lobe epileptics with abnormal aggressivity. He used inlying electrodes to record brain waves and found that his patients experienced frequent electrical seizures in the depths of their brains that were not reflected in surface recordings or in clinical seizure states, thus confirming our observations in Chapter 8. Walker suggested that these subclinical seizures were related to the greater frequency of aggressive behavior occurring between obvious epileptic seizures. Sweet and Mark presented an extensive review of the relationship between aggressive behavior and brain abnormality for the Association for Research in Nervous and Mental Disease.[3]

VIOLENCE AND THE BRAIN focuses on abnormally aggressive individuals whose brain disease has made them objects of legitimate medical concern. Violence, however, can be more than a medical problem. Appendix I outlines our attempt to set the limits, particularly of surgical treatment.[4]

Each of the patients described in detail in Chapters 6, 7 and 8 of this book had previously been reported in the medical literature. The only patient whose surgical treatment was reported in detail was Clara (Ch. 6). Her case was included in a report in the *Transactions of the American Neurological Association*[5] as an example of improved behavior in the presence of persistent seizures. At the present time, over ten years after surgery, she still has the neurological deficit that she had before amygdala surgery. However, Clara continues to function as a housewife. Her seizures have not been cured but her seizure frequency has been drastically reduced from twenty a day to twenty a year. She still gets angry and her husband complains that she is sometimes difficult to live with. However, she has not had a single rage attack in which she has assaulted another individual.

Thomas (Ch. 7) was reported in the *Archives of Neurology.*[6] Although described as a brilliant engineer in the text, this man was considerably disabled by the time of surgery. He had suffered seizures, rage attacks and hallucinations for 14 years. His condition did not respond to years of psychiatric care including three years of psychiatric management under one physician with two years of anticonvulsant therapy. He decompensated especially in the six months preceding surgery and had to be confined in a locked psychiatric ward on one occasion. His behavior before surgery was at times described as "frankly psychotic" (page 93). His postsurgical condition can be summarized as follows: he had had no epileptic seizures for the last three years and only one reported rage attack. However, his periods of confusion and disordered thinking (p. 97) have continued with paranoid delusions and ideas of reference along with hysterical episodes.[7]

A similar thought disorder that develops in epileptic patients has been described by Slater and Beard.[8] It often becomes full blown years after the onset of epilepsy, especially when the epileptic seizures diminish or stop. Some of the patients reported by these investigators have symptoms almost identical to those of our patient Thomas. Observations of behavioral disorders associated with epilepsy have been reconfirmed by Falconer,[9A] with an accompanying editorial by Geschwind,[9B] who suggests that the kind of psychosis described above may be specifically related to epilepsy.

Julia (Ch. 7) had been previously described by Mark *et. al.*[10] Since surgery, her seizure frequency has diminished somewhat and in the last two years, she has not exhibited assaultive behavior. She still has episodes of impulsive anger but this is directed and does not get out of her control. She was institutionalized for several years before surgery and had to continue an institutional life after operation because of her continued psychotic state (p. 108). However, recently, she has been able to live at home, sing in the choir, attend daily adult education classes, and pass her high school equivalency examinations.

Jennie (Ch. 8), suspected of suffering from a brain tumor, had previously been reported.[11] Jennie did not have therapeutic lesions in her brain; she was taken off of anticonvulsant medication against our expressed desires when she left the hospital. Subsequently, she continued to experience repeated episodes of attack behavior directed at young children. These were so extreme and dangerous that she had to be removed to an adult institution.

Most of the patients described in Chapter 9 were part of a population undergoing neurological and psychiatric study by a medical group whose report was subsequently published.[12] All of the surgical patients with inlying brain electrodes were described at the Houston Neurological Symposium.

1. Vaernet, K. and Madsen, A. Lesions in the amygdala and the substantia innominata in aggressive psychotic patients. In: *Psychosurgery* (E. Hitchcock, L. Laitinen and K. Vaernet, eds.) Springfield, Ill., Charles C. Thomas, 1972.
2. Walker, A. E. Man and his temporal lobes: John Hughlings Jackson Lecture. *Surg. Neurol. 1*:69–79, Mar. 1973.
3. Mark, V. H. and Sweet, W. H. The role of limbic brain dysfunction in aggression. In ARNMD proceedings to be published by Williams & Wilkins, Baltimore.
4. Mark, V. H. and Neville, R. Social and ethical implications of brain surgery in aggressive epileptics. *JAMA,* in press.
5. Schwab, R. S., Sweet, W. H., Mark, V. H., Kjellberg, R. N. and Ervin, F. R. Treatment of intractable temporal lobe epilepsy by stereotactic amygdala lesions. *Trans. Am. Neurol. Assoc. 90*:12–19, 1965.
6. Stevens, J. R., Mark, V. H., Ervin, F. R., Pacheco, P. and Suematsu, K. Deep temporal stimulation in man: long latency, long lasting psychological changes. *Arch. Neurol. 21*: 157–169, 1969.
7. Mark, V. H. Deep temporal lobe stimulation and destructive lesions in episodically violent temporal lobe patients. In: *The Neurobiology of Violence* (W. S. Fields and W. H. Sweet, eds.) Springfield, Ill., Charles C. Thomas, in press.
8. Slater, E., Beard, A. W. and Glithero, E. The schizophrenia-like psychoses of epilepsy. *Brit. J. Psychiatry 109*:95–150, 1963.

9A. Falconer, M. A. Temporal lobe resection for epilepsy and behavior abnormalities. *NEJM 289:*451, 1973.

B. Geschwind, N. Effects of temporal lobe surgery on behavior. *NEJM 289:*480, 1973.

10. Mark, V. H., Ervin, F. R., Sweet, W. H., Delgado, J.M.R. Remote telemeter stimulation and recording from implanted temporal lobe electrodes. *Confin. Neurol. 31*:86–93, 1969.
11. Sweet, W. H., Ervin, F. R. and Mark, V. H. The relationship of violent behavior to focal cerebral disease. In: *Aggressive Behaviour* (S. Garattini, E. B. Sigg, eds.) Amsterdam, Excerpta Medica Foundation, 1969, pp. 336–352.
12. Bach-y-Rita, G., Lion, J. R., Climent, C. E. and Ervin, F. R. Episodic dyscontrol: a study of 130 violent patients. *Amer. J. Psychiatry 127*:1473–1478, 1971.
13. Mark, V. H., Barry, H., McLardy, T. and Ervin, F. R. The destruction of both anterior thalamic nuclei in a patient with intractable agitated depression. *J. Nerv. Ment. Dis. 150*:266–272, 1970.

Index

Ablation of brain, 27-29
Abdominal discomfort, before seizures, 60, 70, 93
Acquired brain disease, 55-65
Affect, in epilepsy, 62
Aggression, animal studies of, 33-37
Aggressive instincts, 32, 37
Alcohol, affecting brain, 59, 126, 127-128
Amygdala, 24
  removal of, 28-29
  responses to environmental changes, 27
  stereotactic destruction of, 85-86, 94, 96-97, 107
  stimulation of, 30, 92, 96, 99-107
  target areas in, 92
Anatomy of brain, 16-24
Animal studies, of aggressive behavior, 33-37
Anticonvulsants, use of, 9, 63-64, 87, 94, 98, 121, 128, 129, 158
Aristotle, 139
Assaults, physical, in dyscontrol syndrome, 93, 127-128
Attack behavior, experimental, 30-31
Automatisms, stereotyped, in epilepsy, 63
Automobile accidents, head injuries in, 12
Automobiles, violence with, 3, 93, 127, 129, 131
Awareness, in epilepsy, 61

Bandura, A., 150
Basal ganglia, 24
Behavior, dualistic view of, 138-144
Behavior therapy, 158
Brain damage, causes of, 12
Brain-environment interaction, 7-8, 9-10, 33, 138-144
Brain stem
  function of, 14
  injury to, 57

Brain, stimulation of. *See* stimulation of brain
Bucy, P., 28-29

Causes of brain damage, 12
Causes of violence, 2, 3-5, 149-152
Cerebellum, 20
Cerebrum, 20
Chemical stimulation of brain, 159
Chemotherapy. *See* Anticonvulsants
Children, brain damage in, 56-57
Chromosome abnormalities, 48-50
Cingulum, 24
Cloward, R. A., 149
Coghill, G. E., 139
Control of violence
  dyscontrol syndrome, 125-132
  instinctual mechanisms in, 35, 36-37
  mechanisms in, 31, 108
  in riot situations, 151
  and weak learned behavior, 1, 37, 108
Criminal behavior, electroencephalographic changes with, 136-137
Cultural rules for behavior, and memory function, 142
Culture, affecting brain function, 33
Culture-conflict hypothesis of violence, 149
Cytogenetic abnormalities, 47-50

Decortication, effects of, 28
Definitions, of acceptable and unacceptable violence, 159-160
Delgado, J., 97, 99, 111
Depression, in epilepsy, 62
Descartes, 139
Detection of potential violence, need for, 121, 124, 125, 147, 157-158
Diagnosis, indirect methods of, 125
Downer, J., 29
Drug therapy. *See* Anticonvulsants
Dualistic view of behavior, 138-144
Dyscontrol syndrome, 125-132
  and physical assault, 93, 127-128
  relation to violence, 146-152
  sexual aspects of, 128
  symptoms of, 126
  and traffic violence, 127, 129

Electrical activity in brain, recording of, 27
Electrical stimulation of brain. *See* Stimulation of brain
Electroencephalography, 131, 136
  and criminal behavior, 136-137
Embryology of brain, 16-21
Emotional brain, 24
Encephalitis, 57-58, 97
Endleman, S., 150

Environmental conditions, and brain function, 7-8, 9-10, 33, 138-144
Epilepsy, 8, 56, 60-65, 158
  manifestations of, 61-63
  surgery in, 64, 69-85, 94
  types of, 60
  and violent behavior, 8, 64-65, 71, 108
Epithalamus, 21
Ethology, 33-36
Etiology of brain damage, 12
Experience, affecting brain function, 33

Facial pain, before violent behavior, 93
Ferrier, D., 139
Flight or fight mechanisms, 1, 14
  control of, 24
  in epilepsy, 62
  in human brain, 32
Freud, S., 33
Frontal lobe, 20
  destructive lesion in, 142
Frustration, and aggressive behavior, 149

Ganglia, basal, 24
Gangs, juvenile, studies of, 149-150
Genetic brain disease, 47-50, 55
Gibbs, F. A., 136
Goodall, J., 36
Grand mal epilepsy, 60
Group violence, 151-152

Hallucinations, in epilepsy, 62-63
Head injuries, damage from, 57, 70
Heimberger, R. R., 85
Hereditary brain disease, 47-50
Hidden brain disease, 112-124
Hippocampus, 24
  abnormal recordings from, 115
  and memory, 142
  removal of, 28
  responses to environmental changes, 27
Homicides, studies of, 126-127, 136
Hospitalized patients, compared with prisoners, 130-132
Hyperkinesis, and brain damage, 56-57
Hypothalamus, 21
  destruction of, 29, 86
  stimulation of, 31

Impulse control, poor, 127, 147
  behavior therapy for, 158
  as observed by patients, 8
Incidence
  of brain disease, 5, 12
  of violent behavior, 3, 146
Infections of brain, viral, 57-58
Inherited brain disease, 47-50
Injuries to head, damage from, 57, 70

Instincts
  aggressive, 32, 37
  and control mechanisms, 35, 36-37
  of self-preservation, 1, 14

James, W., 33
Jones, H. M., 159
Juvenile gangs, studies of, 149-150

Klüver, H., 28-29

Learned behavior, weak, and control of violence, 1, 37, 108
Learning, and memory, 140-142
Levy, S., 136
Lilly, J., 36
Limbic brain, 14-16, 21-24
  after decortication, 28
  stimulation of, 30-31
  tumors of, 59
Lobectomy, in epilepsy, 69
Lobes of brain, 20-21
Lorenz, K., 14, 34

Malamud, N., 59
Mass media, affecting behavior, 150-151
Medical aspects of violence, 5-7
Medications, use of. *See* Anticonvulsants
Memory, and learning, 140-142
Menninger, K., 126
Midbrain, 24
  stimulation of, 30-31
Monroe, R., 126
Montagu, A., 34
Mood changes, in epilepsy, 62
Motivation, and behavior, 30
Murderers, studies of, 126-127, 136

Narabayashi, H., 57, 85
Nature-and-nurture controversy, 34
Neocortex, 14-16
  removal of, 28
Newborn, brain damage in, 56
Nuclei, septal, 24

Occipital lobe, 21
Odors, responses to, 16, 35
Ohlin, L. E., 149, 151
Oswald, L. H., 148
Oxygen insufficiency, effects of, 56

Parietal lobe, 21
Perceptual changes, in epilepsy, 61
Petit mal epilepsy, 60
Predatory animals, behavior of, 35, 36
Prediction of violence, need for, 121, 124, 125, 147, 157-158
Preservation of self, instinct for, 1, 14
Prevention of violence, 155-161

Prisoners
  compared with hospitalized patients, 130-132
  electroencephalography of, 136-137
Psychotherapy, 87, 93, 98, 128, 158
Public health problem, violence as, 4, 160

Rabies, 58
Rage behavior
  and epilepsy, 8, 64-65, 71, 108
  surgery affecting. *See* Surgery
Recording of electrical activity, in brain, 27
Rehabilitation, efforts in, 144
Remorse, after violent behavior, 5, 97
Reward-seeking behavior, 30
Riots, studies of, 151-152

Sano, K., 86
Scott, J. P., 34
Self-preservation, instinct of, 1, 14
Self-referred patients, 5, 7-8, 130
Sellen, T., 149
Sensory deprivation, effects of, 143
Septal nuclei, 24
Sexual aspects of dyscontrol syndrome, 128
Sherrington, C., 139
Silverman, D., 136
Social causes of violence, 2, 3-5, 149-150
Speck, R., 4, 148
Spiegel, E. A., 87
Spiegel, J., 151
Stafford-Clark, D., 136
Stereotactic surgery, 29, 64, 69-85, 94
  of amygdala, 85-86, 94, 96-97, 107
  in epilepsy, 64, 69-85, 94
  of hypothalamus, 86
  of thalamus, 86
Stereotyped automatisms, in epilepsy, 63
Stimoceiver, use of, 97, 99, 111
Stimulation of brain, 29-31, 159
  in amygdala, 92, 96, 99-107
  remote, 97, 99, 111
  target areas in, 92
Stop points in brain, affecting performance, 31
Storr, A., 37, 127
Structures of brain, 16-24
  changes in, 6
  damage to, 56-59
Studies of violent persons, need for, 156-158
Subcultures, violent behavior in, 149-150
Suicide attempts, 5, 62, 97, 131
Suppression of violence, mechanisms in, 31, 108
Surgery, 27-29, 158-159
  in epilepsy, 64, 69-85
  frontal lobe, 142
  See also Stereotactic surgery

Target areas in brain, stimulation of, 92

Television, effects of, 150-151
Temporal lobe, 21
  removal of, 28
  tumors of, 59
Temporal lobe epilepsy, 60-63, 158
  and hidden brain disease, 113-124
Tests for prediction of violence, need for, 121, 124, 125, 147, 157-158
Thalamus, 21
  and memory functions, 142
  stereotactic lesions in, 86
Thought changes, in epilepsy, 62
Traffic violence, 3, 93, 127, 129, 131
Treatment methods, evaluation of, 158-159
Trigger areas in brain, 108
Tumors of brain, 58-59

Vaernet, K., 86
Victims of violence, number of, 3, 146
Violence, causes of, 2, 3-5, 149-152
Violence (*continued*)
  control of. *See* Control of violence
Viral infections of brain, 57-58

War, as group violence, 151
Warning signs, before violent behavior, 63, 64, 70, 92, 97, 121, 146, 148
Weak learned behavior, and control of violence, 1, 37, 108
Wertham, F., 150
West, D. J., 127
Whitman, C., 4, 148
Willett, T. C., 127
Winkler, G. E., 136
Wolfgang, M. E., 126, 149

XYY chromosomal pattern, 49-50

Yablonsky, L., 149

Zublin, O., 49
Zuckerman, S., 34

73 74 75 76 77 10 9 8 7 6 5 4 3